DATE DUE

	MAY 0 4 2004	
	MAR 1 2 2008	
MAR 2 2 2011		
	MAR 2 7 2009	
	MAR 2 6 2010	
	MAR 2 0 2009	

Diabetic Retinopathy

Diabetic Retinopathy

PRACTICAL MANAGEMENT

R. JOSEPH OLK, M.D.
Washington University Eye Care Network
Associate Professor of Clinical Ophthalmology and Visual Sciences
Washington University School of Medicine
St. Louis, Missouri

CAROL M. LEE, M.D.
Clinical Assistant Professor
Department of Ophthalmology
New York University School of Medicine
New York, New York

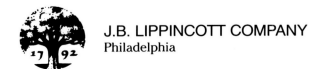

J.B. LIPPINCOTT COMPANY
Philadelphia

Project Editor: Dina Papadopoulos
Indexer: David Amundson
Art Director: Susan Hermansen
Interior and Cover Designer: William T. Donnelly
Production Manager: Caren Erlichman
Production Coordinator: David T. Murphy, Jr.
Compositor: Compset Inc.
Printer/Binder: Arcata Graphics/Kingsport

6   5   4   3   2

Library of Congress Cataloging in Publications Data

Olk, R. Joseph.
    Diabetic retinopathy : practical management / R. Joseph Olk, Carol
M. Lee.
        p.   cm.
    Includes bibliographic references and index.
    ISBN 0-397-51167-1
    1. Diabetic retinopathy.   I. Lee, Carol M.   II. Title.
    [DNLM: 1. Diabetic Retinopathy—therapy.   WK 835 049d]
RE661.D505   1993
617.7′3—dc20
DNLM/DLC
for Library of Congress   92-48876
                                                                                          CIP

I wish to dedicate this book to all of the fellows with whom I have had the privilege of participating in their education and training during the first decade of my own practice (1981–1991). If the quality of the fellows trained in the decade of the 1990s is half as good as those in the decade of the 1980s, I feel I will have been truly blessed. The fellows are as follows:

Harry Engel, 1981–1982	Robert Roseman, 1986–1987
Matthew Lipman, 1981–1982	Lon Poliner, 1986–1987
Greg Mincey, 1982–1983	Linda Margulies, 1986–1987
Stephen Grinde, 1982–1983	Ed Ryan, 1987–1988
Robert Wendel, 1983–1984	Alan Berger, 1987–1989
Michael Feigelman, 1984–1985	Neil Okun, 1988–1989
Clement Chan, 1984–1985	Larry Halperin, 1989–1990
Graham Avery, 1984–1985	Carol Lee, 1989–1991
Brad Jost, 1985–1986	Sam Pesin, 1990–1991
Linda Uniat, 1985–1986	Marc Lowe, 1990–1992

With the training of fellows, I am reminded of the famous quotation delivered by Francis Weld Peabody in a lecture to Harvard Medical students in 1927, and I hope all of these fellows will continue to follow his guiding principles:

"The good physician knows his patients through and through, and his knowledge is bought dearly. Time, sympathy, and understanding must be lavishly dispensed, but the reward is to be found in that personal bond which forms the greatest satisfaction of the practice of medicine. One of the essential qualities of the clinician is interest in humanity, for the secret of the care of the patient is in caring for the patient."

PREFACE

Diabetic Retinopathy: Practical Management presents the cumulative experience of the senior author (R. Joseph Olk, M.D.) over the past decade in diagnosing, managing, and treating patients with diabetic retinopathy. This volume is *not* intended to represent an exhaustive, comprehensive textbook, but rather a succinct, didactic summary of the essentials in evaluating and treating patients with diabetic retinopathy. This book is replete with illustrations that are intended to emphasize the author's treatment techniques. It is obvious that this monograph represents one individual's approach to the management of diabetic retinopathy, and it goes without saying that the authors acknowledge that other diagnostic and therapeutic approaches to the management of diabetic retinopathy are acceptable alternatives as well.

Chapter 1 briefly describes the epidemiology of diabetic retinopathy.

Chapter 2 outlines the classifications of diabetic retinopathy and includes the most recent ETDRS classification of nonproliferative retinopathy.

Chapter 3 updates the results of all of the national collaborative studies involved with the management and treatment of diabetic retinopathy and its complications.

Chapter 4 highlights the management of nonproliferative diabetic retinopathy.

Chapter 5 details the management of diabetic macular edema with special emphasis on the senior author's experience with "modified grid laser photocoagulation."

Chapter 6 discusses the management of proliferative diabetic retinopathy.

Chapter 7 presents indications for vitreous surgery.

Chapter 8 discusses the indications for fluorescein angiography in the management of diabetic retinopathy.

Chapter 9 details the complications and side effects of treatment.

Chapter 10 discusses special cases in the management of patients with various problems associated with diabetic retinopathy, including diabetic retinopathy and cataracts, diabetic macular edema and proliferative retinopathy, diabetic retinopathy and pregnancy, and advanced cases of diabetic macular edema.

It is hoped that *Diabetic Retinopathy* will provide the reader with a basic understanding of the senior author's approach to the management of diabetic patients in everyday clinical practice. Further, we hope that the multitude of illustrations in this text will provide the reader with the in-depth understanding of the various treatment strategies and techniques employed by the senior author so that the ultimate goal of having the patient receive optimum management will have been achieved.

R. Joseph Olk, M.D.
Carol M. Lee, M.D.

ACKNOWLEDGMENTS

A number of individuals have had a significant impact on my professional career over the past decade, especially in regard to diagnosis and management of patients with diabetic retinopathy. It is because of these particular people that I was stimulated to undertake the writing of this book.

First and foremost, my coauthor, Carol M. Lee, has been the most outstanding fellow I have trained to date. Her enthusiasm, industriousness, and attention to detail allowed us to complete this book in a timely fashion.

Arnall Patz, former Department Chairman of the Wilmer Institute at Johns Hopkins Hospital, was the one who encouraged me in 1980–1981 to undertake our pilot study concerning modified grid treatment for diffuse diabetic macular edema.

Stuart Fine, former Director of the Retinal Vascular Center of the Wilmer Institute at Johns Hopkins Hospital and present Chairman of the Department of Ophthalmology at the Scheie Eye Institute in Philadelphia, taught me the true meaning of a "randomized clinical trial." Through his encouragement we were able to conduct our initial as well as many subsequent randomized clinical trials concerning various aspects of management and treatment for diffuse diabetic macular edema.

I wish to thank Nadine Sokol for all of her artist's illustrations, and Emily Chew of the National Eye Institute and Robert Murphy of the Retina Center, St. Joseph's Hospital in Baltimore, for reviewing our chapter on nonproliferative diabetic retinopathy, as well as their invaluable advice.

Lastly, I wish to acknowledge the editorial assistance of Jeanne B. Toma.

CONTENTS

Diabetic Retinopathy

Diabetic Retinopathy: Practical Management, by R. Joseph Olk and Carol M. Lee. J.B. Lippincott Company, Philadelphia © 1993.

CHAPTER · 1

Epidemiology of Diabetic Retinopathy

The clinical importance of timely and appropriate management for diabetic retinopathy rests in the epidemiology of the disease. Diabetic retinopathy is the leading cause of blindness in Americans of working age, 20 to 74 years old, attributing to 12% of all cases of new blindness in 1 year.[1,2] Approximately 700,000 Americans have proliferative retinopathy and 500,000 have macular edema. Approximately 65,000 new cases of proliferative disease and 75,000 new cases of macular edema will occur each year.[2]

Three major national multicenter trials have been established: namely, the Diabetic Retinopathy Study (DRS), Early Treatment Diabetic Retinopathy Study (ETDRS), and Diabetic Retinopathy Vitrectomy Study Research Group (DRVS), each of which has been invaluable in guiding the management of patients with diabetic retinopathy. These and many other studies have demonstrated the statistically significant efficacy of photocoagulation treatment in the management of proliferative diabetic retinopathy and diabetic macular edema. By identifying eyes at high risk for visual loss and applying appropriate treatment, we can intervene in the natural course of diabetic retinopathy with the hope of halting and even reversing the natural progression from its vasoproliferative stage to its fibrotic scarred end stage.

In view of these definitive findings, it is alarming that 55% of eyes with high-risk retinopathy, as defined by the DRS,[3] in the Wisconsin Epidemiologic Study of Diabetic Retinopathy (WESDR) for the prevalence of retinal photocoagulation, had not received photocoagulation treatment.[4] Additionally, in looking at the 4-year incidence of photocoagulation, the WESDR reported that 4 years after initial exam 33% of younger-onset diabetics and 58% of older-onset diabetics with high-risk retinopathy had yet to be treated.[5] Given these numbers and the estimation that 12 million Americans have diabetes,[1,2] it is imperative that all diabetic patients, general practitioners, internists, and ophthalmologists be aware of the importance of recognizing and treating diabetic retinopathy. The Diabetes 2000 program, currently underway, is establishing these goals with both public informational campaigns and educational series for health care workers. We have structured this book along the clinical and practical guidelines for the detection and treatment of diabetic retinopathy.

In all of our chapters, we have used the terminology and clinical classification of diabetic retinopathy established by the ETDRS.[6] This clinically useful scale separates nonproliferative from proliferative retinopathy. Further subdivision separates mild-to-moderate nonproliferative from moderate-to-severe nonproliferative retinopathy based on both clinical findings and the propensity for developing proliferative disease. Proliferative disease is divided into early and high-risk disease. The new classification of mild-to-moderate nonproliferative retinopathy encompasses what traditionally has been called background retinopathy. The classifications of moderate-to-severe and very severe nonproliferative retinopathy incorporate what has traditionally been referred to as preproliferative retinopathy. Their pathophysiologic correlates and significance remain unchanged, but the newer grading scale allows the identification of eyes that have a higher rate of development of proliferative disease and, consequently, severe visual loss, if left untreated. When referring to specific studies, for example, the WESDR, we will use the terminology as used in the original studies.

References

1. National Society to Prevent Blindness. Operational Research Department. Vision problems in the U.S.: a statistical analysis. New York: National Society to Prevent Blindness; 1980:1–46.
2. Patz A, Smith RE. The ETDRS and Diabetes 2000 [Editorial]. Ophthalmology 1991; 98:739–740.
3. Diabetic Retinopathy Study Research Group. DRS report no. 3. Four risk factors for severe visual loss in diabetic retinopathy. Arch Ophthalmol 1979;97: 654–655.
4. Klein R, Klein BEK, Moss SE, Davis MD, DeMets DL. The Wisconsin Epidemiologic Study of Diabetic Retinopathy. VI. Retinal photocoagulation. Ophthalmology 1987; 94:747–753.
5. Klein R, Klein BEK, Moss SE, Davis MD, DeMets DL. The Wisconsin Epidemiologic Study of Diabetic Retinopathy. VIII. The incidence of retinal photocoagulation. Diabetic complications. J Diabetic Complications 1988;2:79–87.
6. Early Treatment Diabetic Retinopathy Study Research Group. ETDRS report no. 12. Fundus photographic risk factors for progression of diabetic retinopathy. Ophthalmology 1991; 98:823–833.

Diabetic Retinopathy: Practical Management, by R. Joseph Olk and Carol M. Lee. J.B. Lippincott Company, Philadelphia © 1993.

CHAPTER · 2

Classification of Diabetic Retinopathy

NONPROLIFERATIVE DIABETIC RETINOPATHY

Early Changes: Mild-to-Moderate Nonproliferative Diabetic Retinopathy

The fundus changes that occur in diabetic retinopathy follow a progressive course from nonproliferative to proliferative. All of the fundus changes described here are a result of diabetic retinal microangiopathy, characterized in its early stages by vascular occlusion and, in its later stages, by fibrovascular proliferation and scar formation.

Both retinal vascular closure causing ischemia and increased retinal vascular permeability are believed to be the main pathophysiologic pathways that cause the fundus changes we have seen clinically. Autopsy specimens of diabetic eyes were first examined in the 1950s with India ink perfusion.[1] In the 1960s, methods using trypsin digestion of the neural tissue were employed that left the vasculature relatively intact.[2] Large areas of capillary nonperfusion were seen to be physically associated with clusters of microaneurysms and to follow the pattern of arteriolar occlusion. Thus, both capillary and arteriolar occlusion appeared to be involved in the development of microaneurysms and other fundus changes.

From studies of capillary wall composition, it also appeared that there was a selective loss of mural pericytes. Some capillaries appeared to have a proliferation of endothelial cells, whereas others lacked any cells—the latter probably representing residual acellular occluded "ghost vessels" with thickened residual basement membrane. Both pericyte loss and thickening of the basement membrane are early changes in the pathologic evolution of diabetes-induced vascular disease.[3] The occlusion of the capillary bed and its intimate association with the fundus changes seen were clearly demonstrated with the development of fluorescein angiography by which areas of nonperfusion could be easily demonstrated.[4–7] The angiographic patterns were correlated histopathologically: the nonperfused capillary bed consisted of acellular strands or cylinders of thickened basement membrane; the hypercellular channels were actually dilated vessels and were well-perfused by fluorescein.

Since retinal vessels are not directly regulated by the autonomic nervous system, autoregulation takes place instead. When there is a relative lack of perfusion, creating a hypoxic condition, retinal vessels will dilate to increase the flow. In diabetic eyes, shortly after the onset of hyperglycemia, microvascular dilation occurs, followed by capillary obliteration and occlusion and microaneurysm formation,[8–11] such that focal areas of capillary closure are often found adjacent to areas of microvascular dilation.[9]

The dilated vessels then may act as shunt vessels, possibly removing even more blood flow from the already compromised retinal areas served by the occluded vessels. Retinal blood flow studies show somewhat contradictory results. Some show that progressive capillary occlusion is associated with an increase in the blood flow through the large retinal vessels.[12,13] Others could detect no change in blood flow by laser Doppler velocimetry. The total flow through the dilated vessels did not contribute to an overall drop in flow, although a decrease in blood flow in the major veins was noted.[14,15]

The macular capillary hemodynamics were studied recently by Sinclair, who found that capillary flow velocity was elevated in diabetic eyes, regardless of the severity of retinopathy, along with a decrease in the density of entoptically perceived leukocytes.[16,17] This may be a psychophysical manifestation of autoregulatory dilation of the microvasculature adjacent to underperfused areas. Later, there is a complete breakdown of the autoregulatory system, whereby the retinal vessels are unable to adequately oxygenate the retinal tissue and, compounded by the vascular occlusion, produce the setting of ischemic retinal tissue.

Microaneurysms

The circulatory changes produce a series of changes seen clinically and referred to in the earlier stages as mild-to-moderate nonproliferative retinopathy (Table 2-1). The first sign is generally the microaneurysm, the location of which indicates areas of capillary closure.[18,19] Microaneurysms appear to derive from retinal capillaries and are usually found in the vicinity of occluded capillaries, as seen both histopathologically and angiographically. Single micro-

TABLE 2–1

"Mild-to-Moderate" Nonproliferative Retinopathy

Microaneurysms
Intraretinal hemorrhages: mild to moderate in fewer than four quadrants
Hard exudates
Macular edema
Foveal avascular zone abnormalities

aneurysms can be found, however, without demonstrable nonperfusion. Microaneurysms can occur at any level between the superficial and deeper retinal capillary networks or even from the choroidal circulation.[20]

Microaneurysms can be from 12 to 100 μm in diameter, but only those larger than 30 μm in diameter are clinically visible.[21,22] The recent Early Treatment Diabetic Retinopathy Study (ETDRS)-grading system, which is an "extension of the Modified Airlie House Classification," gave an upper limit of 125 μm for the diameter and the requirement of sharp margins for a lesion to be considered a microaneurysm. Any red spot larger than 125 μm is considered to be a hemorrhage, unless its characteristics, such as distinct round shape, smooth borders, and central light reflex, are specifically consistent with features of microaneurysms.[23] They appear as bright red spots, but may appear yellowish as their endothelial linings may proliferate with subsequent occlusion and hyalinization of their cavities.[2,3] These small aneurysms may reflect a weakening of the capillary wall in local areas, with loss of pericyte support, causing an outpouching from the capillary wall.[2] They may also represent an active cellular response to retinal hypoxic insult.[19]

More microaneurysms are visible angiographically than clinically, since the smallest ones may be seen only with fluorescein, and the partially occluded ones that are not distinct ophthalmoscopically may fluoresce. Generally, microaneurysms fill during the early venous stage and either retain their size, shape, and dye, or leak as the study progresses. They may surround cotton-wool spots or be surrounded by circinate rings of hard exudates, showing that their presence is due to a vascu-

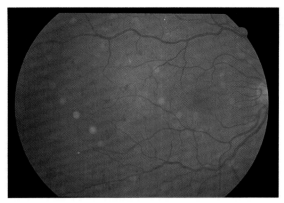

Figure 2–1 This is an example of mild nonprolifera-tive diabetic retinopathy. Microaneurysms are scattered throughout the fundus and temporal to the foveal avas-cular zone, as well as dot-and-blot hemorrhages and a few areas of intraretinal lipid.

lopathy of the retinal vessels. Capillary closure is often visible directly near clusters of micro-aneurysms (Figs. 2-1 and 2-2).

The Foveal Avascular Zone

As mentioned, capillary closure is one of the primary steps in the pathogenesis of diabetic retinopathy. The perifoveal capillary bed can be studied angiographically and can vividly demonstrate capillary occlusion and obliter-

ation. Normally, the foveal avascular zone (FAZ) is clearly seen with fluorescein angiog-raphy. The concentration of underlying mela-nin is highest here, adding to the contrast between the fluorescein-filled capillaries and background choroidal fluorescence. The reti-nal capillary bed is a monolayer at this point, where individual capillaries and their abnor-malities are clearly visible.[19,24] Normally, the foveal avascular zone is approximately 350 to 750 µm in diameter[24,25]; however, this is vari-able. In diabetic eyes, abnormalities of the foveal avascular zone are seen. These abnor-malities include irregular margins, capillary budding into the foveal avascular zone, and widening of the intercapillary spaces within the perifoveolar capillary bed.[24] Bridging ves-sels are noted between areas of capillary drop-out, and the entire diameter and extent of the foveal avascular zone enlarges. Some capillar-ies appear dilated and are more clearly seen, especially when contrasted with the areas of relative hypofluorescence owing to nonperfu-sion. Again, this dilation is an autoregulatory response to the adjacent hypoperfused and rel-atively hypoxic retinal tissue.

Bresnick has shown that visual acuity is usu-ally diminished when the dimensions of the foveal avascular zone are greater than 1000 µm in longest diameter.[24] However, functional cor-

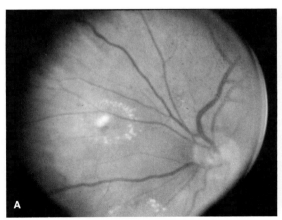
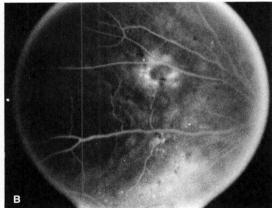

Figure 2–2 **(A,B)** An example of mild-to-moderate nonproliferative diabetic retinopathy, with a circinate ring of hard exudate surrounding microaneurysms. Note that in the fluorescein angiogram **(B)** there is leakage from the microaneurysms and that there is no blocking defect from the hard exudates. Within the circinate ring, there is a small area of blockage secondary to a blot hemor-rhage.

relation is difficult because the foveal avascular zone of a normal eye may have, as an upper limit, up to 1000 μm in diameter, and one cannot predict with accuracy the visual acuity based solely on the appearance of the FAZ.

Intraretinal Hemorrhages

Intraretinal hemorrhages may appear secondary to ruptured microaneurysms, capillaries, or venules. Their shape is dependent on their location within the retinal layers. Dot hemorrhages, with very distinct borders, and blot hemorrhages, with somewhat fuzzier borders, are located deeper within the outer plexiform and inner nuclear layers. Since there is a looser arrangement of cells in these deeper layers, the hemorrhages can take on the shapes of the looser extracellular space. Dot hemorrhages can be distinguished from microaneurysms by fluorescein angiography. Whereas microaneurysms are usually hyperfluorescent, dot hemorrhages (as well as all other intraretinal hemorrhages) block fluorescein and appear as hypofluorescent spots.

Flame-shaped hemorrhages occur in the superficial nerve fiber layer; here, the tighter organization of the cells and the relative paucity of extracellular space allow the hemorrhage to follow the configuration of the nerve fibers or axons (Fig. 2-3). Some hemorrhages have a white center, probably representing autoocclusion if the source of the hemorrhage was a mi-

croaneurysm. Or the center may contain platelets or fibrin; these generally do not herald such grave diseases as systemic bacteremia or other conditions usually associated with white-centered hemorrhages.[26]

Intraretinal hemorrhages usually resolve in 6 weeks to 3 to 4 months without visual obscuration, unless the hemorrhages are located within the fovea. These hemorrhages are usually scattered throughout the posterior pole, but can be seen anywhere, including only in the periphery. If only peripheral hemorrhages are seen, or mainly only nerve fiber layer hemorrhages are seen, other etiologies should be considered. For instance, in the former, causes of peripheral vascular occlusive disease, such as sarcoidosis, should be considered; in the latter, vein occlusion should be considered, in addition to diabetes.

Hard Exudates

Hard exudates are often seen in either individual streaks or clusters or in large circinate rings surrounding clusters of microaneurysms. These are usually located within the outer plexiform layer and glisten, appearing waxy or yellowish-white. The exudate is made up of serum lipoproteins, thought to leak from the abnormally permeable blood vessels,[27] especially across the walls of leaking microaneurysms. Hard exudates also can be seen scattered anywhere in the posterior pole, but they have an affinity for the macula, being intimately associated with retinal thickening.[27–30] In certain cases, hard exudate may deposit subretinally, causing photoreceptor degeneration; this will be visually significant if located within the fovea.

Hard exudates can be reabsorbed either spontaneously or following laser photocoagulation,[28–31] being phagocytosed by macrophages. However, hard exudates present chronically may organize into hard plaques, eventually forming a disciform-type scar.[32] On fluorescein angiography, hard exudate generally does not block fluorescence unless very heavy thick plaques occur; on red-free photography, the hard exudate will be easily visible (Figs. 2-4 and 2-5).

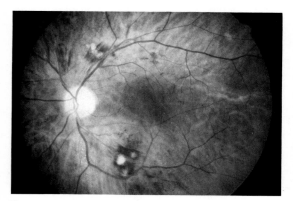

Figure 2–3 An example of mild-to-moderate nonproliferative disease with nerve fiber layer hemorrhage, dot-and-blot hemorrhage, and cotton-wool spots.

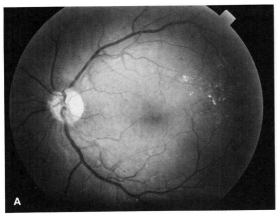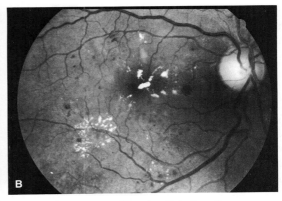

Figure 2–4 These two examples demonstrate mild-to-moderate nonproliferative diabetic retinopathy. (**A**) Hard exudate and microaneurysms are seen temporal to the macula. (**B**) Dot-and-blot hemorrhage, scattered exudate, some in circinate pattern, and early clinically significant macular edema are seen. Note also one intraretinal cotton-wool spot just above the foveal avascular zone.

Macular Edema

Macular edema, the most common cause of decreased vision in patients with nonproliferative retinopathy,[28,29,33] is caused partly by dysfunction at the level of the inner blood–retinal barrier. Abnormally permeable retinal capillary endothelial cells[28,29] of microaneurysms, capillaries, and intraretinal microvascular abnormalities (IRMA) cause leakage of serum lipoproteins and other plasma constituents, which

accumulate in the extracellular space. Although fluorescein leakage is often visible in macular edema, macular edema is clinically defined only when retinal thickening is noted on slit-lamp biomicroscopy during the clinical examination, either with a contact or hand-held lens.

Two distinct types of macular edema have been described: focal and diffuse.[28,29] Focal macular edema derives from individual microaneurysms or small clusters of microaneu-

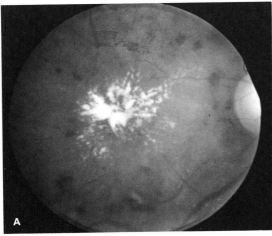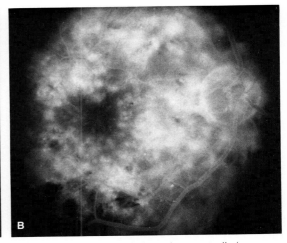

Figure 2–5 An example of exudative maculopathy. (**A**) Note the dense hard exudate centrally in the fovea in a stellate pattern. (**B**) A late-frame fluorescein angiogram shows diffuse leakage from the posterior pole capillary bed. The hard exudate does not block fluorescein, although in cases with extensive exudate, fluorescein blockage may occur.

rysms that histopathologically leak in a more limited extent. These microaneurysms are usually seen in association with streaks or spots of hard exudate or with strictly delineated circinate hard exudate rings (Fig. 2-6). Diffuse macular edema, on the other hand, derives from extensively damaged capillaries, microaneurysms, and arterioles in a capillary bed that appears to be generally dilated. Again, the dilation is assumed to be an autoregulatory response to the adjacent occluded or partially perfused vessels. These dilated vessels have extremely hyperpermeable walls and leak copious amounts of fluid (Figs. 2-7 and 2-8).

Cystoid macular edema often accompanies diffuse macular edema because the outer plexiform and inner nuclear layers are overwhelmed by the large amounts of extracellular fluid (Fig. 2-9). The outer blood–retinal barrier may also be affected in diffuse diabetic macular edema, whereby abnormal retinal pigment epithelial cells are unable to maintain their normal pump functions for the extracellular and subretinal space, as seen experimentally in the streptozocin-induced diabetic animals.[34]

Clinically, a combination of both focal leakage and diffuse leakage is usually seen; this pattern of leakage can be determined by fluorescein angiography. However, the diagnosis of macular edema is made on the basis of clinically observed retinal thickening and not by angiography. In practice, we obtain a fluorescein angiogram, once the decision to treat the macular edema has been made, to help in the determination of vascular perfusion as well as the pattern and type of treatment.

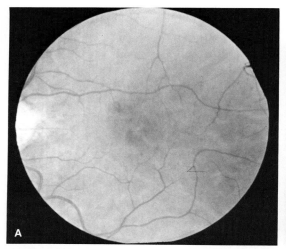

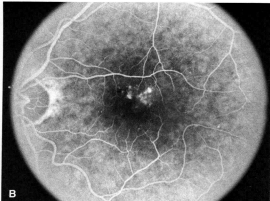

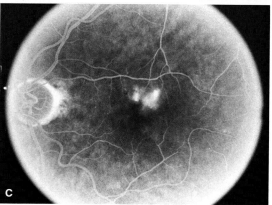

Figure 2–6 A 74-year-old white man with adult-onset insulin-dependent diabetes presented with visual acuity of 20/25 in his left eye with (**A**) early clinically significant macular edema and no evidence of proliferative disease and retinal thickening within 500 μm of the center of the macula associated with microaneurysms. (**B**) Fluorescein angiography showed punctuate spots of hyperfluorescence in the early frames. (**C**) Late frames showed leakage superior to the FAZ in the area of microaneurysms. This is an example of macular edema secondary to focal leakage. It was felt that this patient would benefit from focal laser photocoagulation to areas of leakage in the paramacular region to stabilize his central acuity within the ETDRS guidelines.

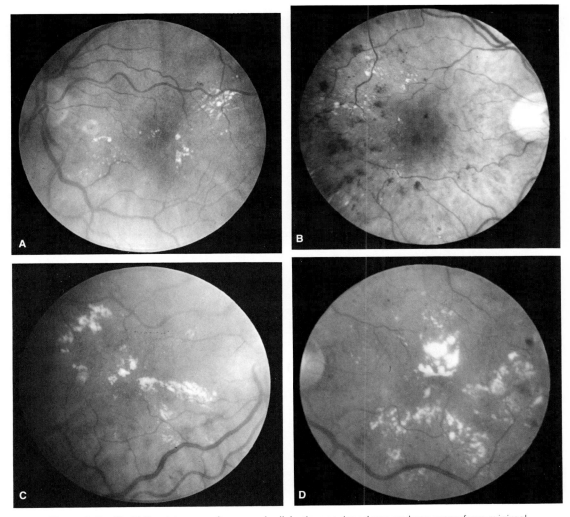

Figure 2–7 (**A–D**) Exudates are often seen in diabetic macular edema and can range from minimal exudate to more extensive involvement.

The foregoing clinical findings of microaneurysms, intraretinal hemorrhages, hard exudates, macular edema, and FAZ abnormalities constitute what was previously referred to as background diabetic retinopathy and what we now prefer to call mild-to-moderate nonproliferative diabetic retinopathy.[23,35–38] However, the severity of the microaneurysms and intraretinal hemorrhages may move the grading of an eye into the more advanced stages of severe and very severe nonproliferative retinopathy as will be discussed in Chapter 4.[23,35,38]

Later Changes: Moderate-to-Severe Nonproliferative Diabetic Retinopathy

As the retina becomes more severely affected by the processes of vascular occlusion and increased vascular permeability, nonproliferative retinopathy worsens. The spectrum of changes that will be described in the following section incorporates findings consistent with what was previously called preproliferative disease and is now defined as moderate-to-

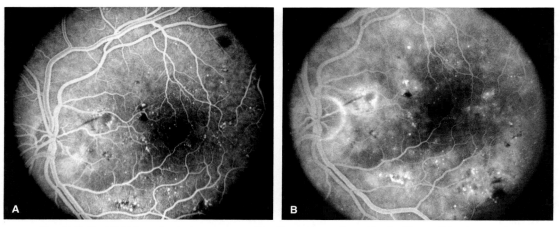

Figure 2–8 (**A**) This patient shows nonproliferative retinopathy with significant diabetic macular edema in the left eye. Fluorescein angiography revealed diffuse leakage from the perifoveal capillary network and enlargement of the FAZ. Early (**A**), late (**B**).

severe nonproliferative diabetic retinopathy (Table 2-2). The presence and severity of these clinical characteristics will determine the level of nonproliferative disease at which an eye can be placed. The division of nonproliferative disease between mild, moderate, severe, and very severe is a useful clinical scale in attempting to predict which eyes will advance to proliferative retinopathy.

Cotton-Wool Spots or Soft Exudates

More advanced nonproliferative retinopathy is heralded by extensive arteriolar closure and is clinically manifest in cotton-wool spots, dot-and-blot hemorrhages, and venous beading.[39,40] Cotton-wool spots, or soft exudates, are actually small infarcts of the nerve fiber layers. They are created by either occlusion or by a transient decrease in flow of an arteriole, with consequent axoplasmic stasis and swelling in the retinal tissue supplied by this arteriole. Soft exudates are seen as fluffy white spots, often marked by the striations of the nerve fiber layer (Fig. 2-10).

Dot-and-blot hemorrhages are the result of hemorrhagic retinal infarcts; these are likely caused by arteriolar occlusion, with later re-

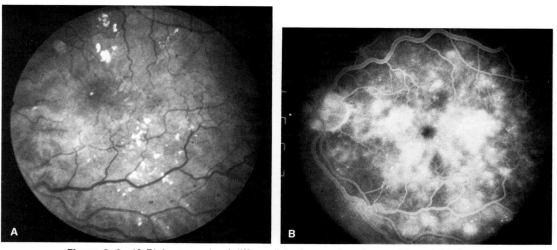

Figure 2–9 (**A,B**) An example of diffuse diabetic macular edema with cystoid change.

TABLE 2–2
"Moderate-to-Severe" Nonproliferative Retinopathy

Cotton-wool spots

Intraretinal hemorrhages: mild to moderate in four quadrants

Venous beading

Intraretinal microvascular abnormalities (IRMA)

perfusion of the arteriole.[19] Fluorescein angiography shows early blockage of fluorescein by the cotton-wool spot or dark blot hemorrhage and is generally associated with zones of capillary nonperfusion surrounding an occluded terminal arteriole.[5] The occluded arteriole may cause remodeling of the capillary bed, with a resultant picture of occluded terminal vessels, new budding capillaries into areas of nonperfusion, and microaneurysms. These may all leak fluorescein late in the angiogram.

Cotton-wool spots are seen in many other diseases, including vein occlusions, carotid artery obstruction, collagen vascular disorders, and cytomegalovirus retinitis. They generally resolve in 2 to 3 months,[41] although it may take much longer (up to a year), leaving an abnormal light reflex at the original site. This represents residual atrophy of the nerve fiber layer and ganglion cells where the cotton-wool spot once was present, and it is referred to as a retinal *depression sign*.[42] Additionally, a rapid in-

crease in the number of cotton-wool spots is seen after patients are brought under strict "tight" metabolic control. Pathophysiologically, this may show that an insult or change to the metabolic milieu, as well as vascular occlusion, can precipitate the formation of cotton-wool spots.[43–45]

Venous Beading

Cotton-wool spots are often found in intimate apposition to areas of both arteriolar and capillary nonperfusion and venous beading. Venous beading represents focal areas of venous dilatation with apparent thinning of the venous wall. Other venous abnormalities include loops of veins sometimes in the shape of an omega (Ω) symbol and reduplication of a venous segment, in addition to venous sheathing and focal narrowing (Fig. 2-11). These changes are associated with capillary nonperfusion and retinal ischemia and are definitely correlated with an increased probability of progression to proliferative retinopathy.[38] Histopathologically, the walls of the beaded veins eventually become thickened and undergo hyaline degeneration.

Intraretinal Microvascular Abnormalities

Intraretinal microvascular abnormalities (IRMA) is a general term used to describe the overall

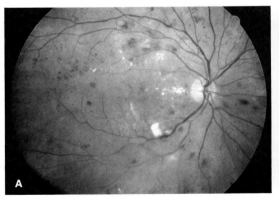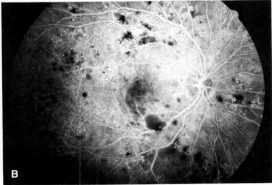

Figure 2–10 (**A,B**) An example of nonproliferative diabetic retinopathy with peripheral ischemia. Note that the cotton-wool spot along the inferotemporal arcade is associated with capillary nonperfusion. Scattered about the posterior pole are intraretinal exudates, dot-and-blot hemorrhages, and nerve fiber layer hemorrhages. Mild venous beading is seen along the supertemporal veins.

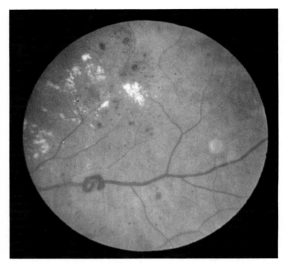

Figure 2–11 Vascular abnormalities in nonproliferative disease can take many shapes and forms. This is an example of one change that has been described as an omega loop.

pathologic changes that occur in the diseased capillary bed and refer specifically to the dilated, tortuous telangiectatic channels that occur between diseased arterioles and venules.[23,46,47] These dilated capillary channels are present within areas of arteriolar and capillary nonperfusion and appear as fine blood-filled vessels. Intraretinal microvascular abnormalities are sometimes difficult to differentiate from early surface neovascularization; although both can leak fluorescein, IRMA do not show the same degree of profuse leakage as do neovascular fronds. The IRMA may also represent intraretinal neovascularization, as described by Muraoka.[47] Intraretinal neovascularizations are believed to be new collateralized vessels within nonperfused retina, deriving from a retinal venule and developing new capillary loops, which also drain into a retinal venule. These new vessels, or channels, have only minimal dye leakage and may be an attempt by the retinal vessels to repair the damaged capillary bed with new channels. These abnormalities are all probably a continuum of pathologic changes in response to the capillary nonperfusion that is present. Similar to venous beading, IRMA are associated with an increased

risk of developing proliferative changes[23,38] (Fig. 2-12).

The clinical findings described thus far constitute nonproliferative changes. The extended version of the modified Airlie House Classification as reported by the ETDRS is used, along with the statistical evidence that any single factor is predictive of progression to more severe disease, to produce a severity scale. This severity scale can then be used to differentiate mild, moderate, severe, and very severe nonproliferative change[23,35–38] (Tables 2-3 and 2-4). For instance, although it has been believed that soft exudates might be especially predictive for the development of proliferative retinopathy,[39,40] the ETDRS found that the predictive power of the presence and severity of venous beading, IRMA, and severe hemorrhages or microaneurysms had a higher association with the development of proliferative disease at the 1-, 3-, and 5-year follow-up visits.[38] In fact, venous beading was the most powerful individual predictor for the risk of future proliferative disease when compared with all other individual factors. Cotton-wool spots were found not to have significant predictive power when compared with the other individual factors.[38] In the ETDRS, hard and soft exudates, without the coexistence of IRMA, venous beading, or severe microaneurysms or intraretinal hemorrhages, or a combination thereof, did not significantly increase the rate of progression of retinopathy.[38]

Midperipheral Ischemia

The importance of the location of arteriolar occlusion is shown in the superwide field fluorescein angiographic studies by Shimizu et al.[48,49] They demonstrated that the midperipheral retina appears to undergo far more capillary nonperfusion than the posterior retina and that midperipheral nonperfusion is highly associated with neovascularization of the disc, retina, and angle (Fig. 2-13). Although it appears that arteriolar and capillary nonperfusion of the posterior pole does not produce a higher rate of neovascularization, posterior pole ischemia, especially of the macula, can produce significant functional impairment.

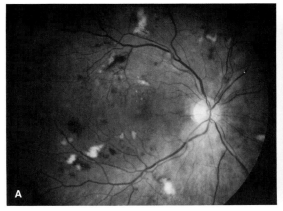

Figure 2–12 An example of extensive severe non-proliferative diabetic retinopathy in a 58-year-old white woman. (**A**) The fundus photograph reveals scattered cotton-wool spots and dot-and-blot hemorrhages, with obvious vascular abnormalities. (**B**) The fluorescein angiogram shows areas of capillary nonperfusion scattered about the posterior pole with vascular remodeling, venous beading, and capillary blunting. The foveal avascular zone is irregular and enlarged. (**C**) In the late frame of the angiogram the areas of venous abnormalities and IRMA stain, but do not appear to leak late. There is one area, however, superotemporal to the fovea, adjacent to an area of capillary nonperfusion that leaks and may be consistent with early surface NVE. There is diffuse leakage of the parafoveal capillary bed.

Although the perfusion of the retina can be determined only angiographically, the markedly ischemic retina will appear whiter and duller than a normal retina. Sheathing of both the larger arteries and veins may be present and, as there is no perfusion, the markedly ischemic retina is usually devoid of hemorrhages, microaneurysms, and hard exudates—otherwise described as "featureless." Other changes that arterioles can undergo include focal narrowing, sheathing, obliteration of their end terminals, and pruning of the arterial tree—all best seen with angiography. Increased permeability through the damaged arteriolar wall will be noted as fluorescein staining.

Although the angiographic characteristics are important in correlating the pathophysiology with the level of retinopathy and in determining the extent of the perfusion or nonperfusion of the capillary bed, clinically, the angiogram is of minimal practical significance

TABLE 2–3
"Severe" Nonproliferative Retinopathy (ETDRS)

Any one of the following:
- Severe intraretinal hemorrhages in four quadrants
- Venous beading in two quadrants
- Moderately severe IRMA in one quadrant

TABLE 2–4
"Very Severe" Nonproliferative Retinopathy (ETDRS)

Any two of the following:
- Severe intraretinal hemorrhages in four quadrants
- Venous beading in two quadrants
- Moderately severe IRMA in one quadrant

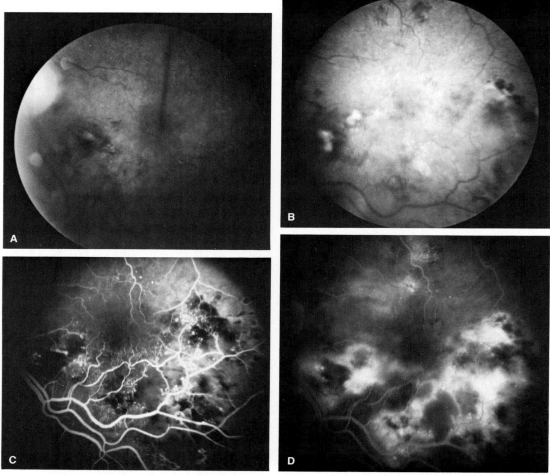

Figure 2–13 (**A,B**) This 81-year-old black woman with non–insulin-dependent diabetes for 20 years is an example of severe nonproliferative diabetic retinopathy with increasing ischemia of the posterior pole and periphery. Fluorescein characteristics of nonproliferative changes are shown: there are marked capillary abnormalities with venous beading and an enlarged foveal avascular zone. (**C,D**) The vessels that traversed the ischemic zone stain late. Visual acuity is 20/200.

in the classification of retinopathy, since findings of nonproliferative and proliferative disease are well correlated both by clinical ophthalmoscopy and fundus photography.

PROLIFERATIVE DIABETIC RETINOPATHY

The hallmark of proliferative diabetic retinopathy is *neovascularization*—new blood vessels that arise from the retina and optic disc and proliferate along the retinal surface or into the vitreous with or without a fibrous component[50] (Table 2-5). Numerous theories have been postulated about the pathogenesis and etiology of the factors influencing the development of new vessels. Vasoproliferative growth factors, inhibitory factors, and chronic hyperglycemia, as well as the enzymatic and nonenzymatic pathways of glucose metabolism, may play a role in the development of diabetic retinopathy. An excellent review by Frank provides references for these numerous studies and hypotheses beyond the scope of this chapter.[51]

TABLE 2–5
Proliferative Retinopathy

Neovascularization of the disc
Neovascularization of the retina elsewhere
Preretinal hemorrhage
Vitreous hemorrhage
Tractional retinal detachment
Neovascularization of the iris or angle, or both

Neovascularization

The nonproliferative changes already described, when accompanied by significant capillary and arteriolar nonperfusion and abnormal permeability, will usually progress to proliferative retinopathy. Neovascularization is most commonly associated with midperipheral capillary nonperfusion[48] and is most commonly located posteriorly within 45° of the optic disc and, especially, on the optic disc itself.[48–50,52] Neovascularization of the disc (NVD) appears as fine wisps or strands of blood vessels, sometimes looping across other disc vessels. They appear to bud off earlier more proximal loops, creating an apparent advancing edge.[21] Early NVD is best appreciated with a contact lens, such as Goldmann; a posterior pole lens; a noncontact magnified lens, such as a Hruby; or a 60-, 78-, or 90-diopter hand-held lens. Direct ophthalmoscopy using the red-free filter can also be useful. If any doubt exists, despite careful clinical examination and stereo color fundus photography, angiography or angioscopy can show the neovascularization clearly, because these new vessels leak dye profusely (Fig. 2-14).

In the Diabetic Retinopathy Study (DRS), NVD is defined as new vessels located on or within one disc diameter of the optic disc[53]; this terminology is maintained here. All other neovascularization is referred to as neovascularization elsewhere, or NVE.

Neovascularization elsewhere is seen as a wheel-like network of fine vessels, usually arising from the retinal veins, venules, or capillaries, and crossing between the arterial and venous sides. They are most readily appreciated with a combination of indirect binocular ophthalmoscopy and direct ophthalmoscopy. Because subtle NVE may be difficult to see

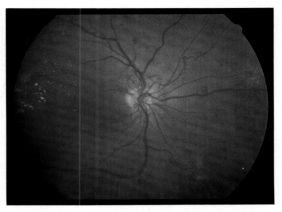

Figure 2–14 An example of neovascularization of the disc (NVD).

clinically, stereo fundus photographs using the seven standard fields of the modified Airlie House Classification can be a useful adjunct.[23,53] In comparison with IRMA, NVE usually occupies a slightly more anterior position in front of the retina, best appreciated with slit-lamp biomicroscopy, aided by a contact lens or hand-held biconvex lens. Although originating intraretinally, NVE will eventually break through the retinal internal limiting membrane to proliferate and extend between the internal limiting membrane and posterior hyaloid face[54] (Figs. 2-15 and 2-16).

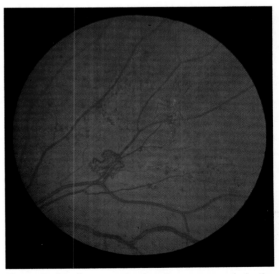

Figure 2–15 An example of surface neovascularization elsewhere (NVE).

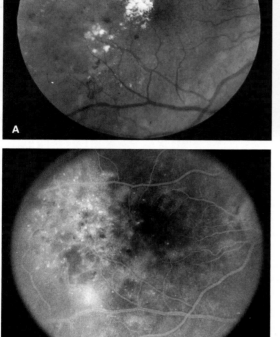

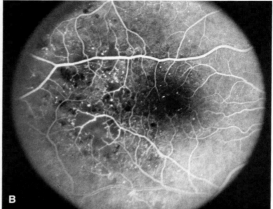

Figure 2–16 An example of diffuse diabetic macular edema with late nonproliferative and early proliferative changes. (**A**) Note the hard exudate in the macula and the NVE inferotemporally. (**B**) On fluorescein angiography, there is capillary nonperfusion and venous beading. (**C**) In the late frame of the angiogram, there is diffuse diabetic macular edema temporal to the foveal avascular zone and leakage from the surface NVE inferotemporally.

Hemorrhage

New vessels are often adherent to the posterior hyaloid. This is clearly seen when a posterior vitreous detachment occurs, elevating the edges of the adherent neovascular complex. Before the posterior vitreous detachment, the neovascular complex generally lies on the surface or only slightly anterior to the retina.

It is the intimate dependence of the fibrovascular and neovascular tissue, which use the posterior hyaloid as a scaffold for further growth and extension, that will determine whether the new vessels will progress to cause hemorrhage and tractional detachment. Neovascularization of the disc rarely develops in an eye that has undergone a complete poste-

rior vitreous detachment or has undergone total vitrectomy with removal of the posterior hyaloid.

New vessels with their adhesions to the posterior vitreous will often hemorrhage as a posterior vitreous detachment occurs. Vitreous traction on these delicate new vessels causes the bleeding, and the blood will often be trapped between the retina and detaching posterior hyaloid in the preretinal or subhyaloid space in a classic boat-like configuration. This configuration delineates the portion of attached to detached vitreous relative to the retinal surface (Figs. 2-17, 2-18, and 2-19). The posterior vitreous is pulled forward by the detachment itself. The contraction of the neovascular tissue growing along the posterior hy-

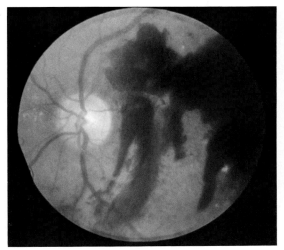

Figure 2–17 An example of preretinal hemorrhage obscuring much of the posterior pole. This was associated with mild NVD as well as NVE.

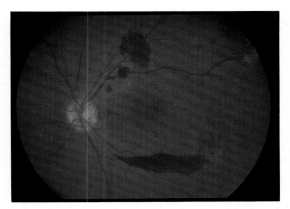

Figure 2–19 An example of proliferative diabetic retinopathy with NVD, boat-shaped preretinal hemorrhage along the inferotemporal arcade, preretinal hemorrhage along the superotemporal arcade, and preretinal fibrosis temporally.

aloid surface also pulls the entire complex forward and exerts more traction along the still attached vitreoretinal adhesive points.

Blood can break through the posterior hyaloid or internal limiting membrane into the vitreous. The blood eventually is resorbed, although large thick hemorrhages can be quite slow to resorb, taking longer than a year if left to their own course. The posterior vitreous is often thickened at its points of attachment to the retinal vessels and fibrovascular proliferations. The detached posterior vitreous may

have varying layers of thickness along its extent, occasionally dotted by hemorrhage and zones of fibrous tissue. These features are visible with careful slit-lamp biomicroscopy. Lastly, the vitreous may detach peripherally, but its tight connections to NVD often preclude total detachment.

Tractional Retinal Detachment

As NVD and NVE progress, fibrous proliferations develop that become entangled within the new vessels and are also adherent to the posterior vitreous face. With increasing proliferation, the fibrovascular complex extends from the disc along the arcades, especially temporally, and often forms a ring connecting the disc with the superotemporal to the inferotemporal arcade. The traction exerted parallel to the retina by the fibrovascular tissue is called *tangential traction.*[54–56] If this fibrovascular mass undergoes significant contraction and if the tightest vitreoretinal adhesions are located on the disc, the macula itself may be dragged, usually, toward the disc.[57] Posterior vitreous detachment here can cause a tabletop configuration of retinal detachment, with the macula detached and with residual points of adhesion in a circle along the arcades (Fig. 2-20).

As the fibrovascular component proliferates and contracts and as the vitreous gel contracts

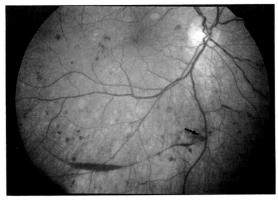

Figure 2–18 An example of proliferative diabetic retinopathy with NVE and a preretinal boat-shaped hemorrhage. Note the tuft of NVE along a branch of the inferotemporal vein (*arrow*).

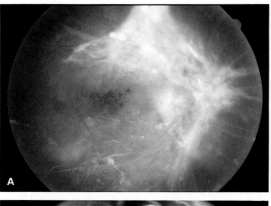

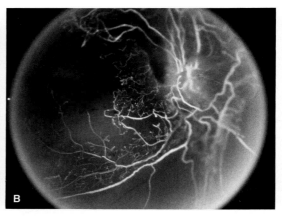

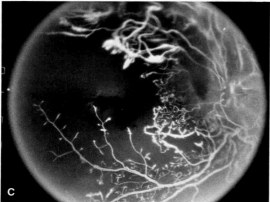

Figure 2–20 A 55-year-old black man with insulin-dependent diabetes of 30-years duration presented with visual acuity of count fingers, having never seen an ophthalmologist. He is seen with a tractional retinal detachment of the posterior pole with significant fibrosis, sclerosis of the blood vessels, and end-stage proliferative diabetic retinopathy. (**A**) There are flecks of preretinal blood overlying the macula. Fluorescein angiography demonstrated marked ischemia to the entire retina. (**B,C**) Note the remodeling of the remaining vasculature, with collateralization of the residual capillaries in the posterior pole. The blockage in the foveal area is secondary to the preretinal hemorrhage, as seen in (**A**).

with progressive posterior detachment, some eyes will undergo tractional retinal detachment. The location of the detachment varies; the majority remain extramacular. However, progressive macular detachment can be seen in up to 14% of cases in 1 year and up to 23% in 3 years.[58] Rarely, an eye may undergo complete spontaneous posterior vitreous detachment, releasing the retinal traction, resulting in spontaneous reattachment of the retina.

The proliferating new vessels will eventually regress if left to their natural course.[54,59,60] The new vessels themselves will become fibrotic. They appear sheathed at first, until the vessels become completely occluded and are replaced by an avascular glial scar tissue mass. This is referred to as *involutional* or *end-stage retinopathy,* or "burnt out" retinopathy, and is accompanied by attenuated vessels and a pale optic disc. If the new vessels and their fibrous proliferations are not subject to vitreous or fi-

brovascular contraction, they may progress from new vessels through the fibrovascular stage, to the involutional-scarring stage, without tractional detachment or vitreous hemorrhage. Our goal is to try to halt this natural progression of disease with timely treatment before the development of the active fibrovascular stage of diabetic retinopathy (Table 2-6).

TABLE 2–6
High-Risk Retinopathy (DRS)

Any three of the following:
- Presence of new vessels
- Location of new vessels on the disc
- Severity of new vessels
    If NVD ≥ one-quarter to one-third disc area or
    standard photograph 10A
    If NVE ≥ one-half disc area
    If both NVD and NVE, count severity of NVD
- Presence of preretinal or vitreous hemorrhage

References

1. Ashton N. Injection of the retinal vascular system in the enucleated eye in diabetic retinopathy. Br J Ophthalmol 1950; 34:38–41.
2. Cogan DG, Toussaint D, Kuwabara T. Retinal vascular patterns. IV. Diabetic retinopathy. Arch Ophthalmol 1961; 66:366–378.
3. Yanoff M. Diabetic retinopathy. N Engl J Med 1966; 274:1344–1349.
4. Kohner EM, Dollery CT, Paterson JW, et al. Arterial fluorescein studies in diabetic retinopathy. Diabetes 1967; 16:1–10.
5. Kohner E, Henkind P. Correlation of fluorescein angiogram and retinal digest in diabetic retinopathy. Am J Ophthalmol 1970; 69:403–410.
6. Cunha-Vaz JG. Diabetic retinopathy. Human and experimental studies. Trans Ophthalmol Soc UK 1972; 92:111–124.
7. Bresnick GH, Engerman R, Davis MD, et al. Patterns of ischemia in diabetic retinopathy. Trans Am Acad Ophthalmol Otolaryngol 1976; 81:694.
8. Bohlen HG, Hankins KD. Early arteriolar and capillary changes in streptozotocin-induced diabetic rats and intraperitoneal hyperglycemic rats. Diabetologia 1982; 22:344–348.
9. Stefansson E, Landers MB III, Wolbarsht ML. Oxygenation and vasodilation in relation to diabetic and other proliferative retinopathies. Ophthalmic Surg 1983; 14:209–226.
10. Zatz R, Brenner BM. Pathogenesis of diabetic microangiopathy. The hemodynamic view. Am J Med 1986; 80:443–453.
11. Small KW, Stefansson E, Hatchell DL. Retinal blood flow in normal and diabetic dogs. Invest Ophthalmol Vis Sci 1987; 28:672–675.
12. Kohner EM, Hamilton AM, Saunders SJ. The retinal blood flow in diabetes. Diabetologia 1975; 11:27–33.
13. Cunha-Vaz JG, Fonseca JR, de Abreau JRF, et al. Studies on retinal blood flow. II. Diabetic retinopathy. Arch Ophthalmol 1978; 96:809–811.
14. Yoshida A, Feke GT, Morales-Stoppello J, et al. Retinal blood flow alterations during progression of diabetic retinopathy. Arch Ophthalmol 1983; 101:225–227.
15. Grunwald JE, Riva CE, Sinclair SH, et al. Laser Doppler velocimetry study of retinal circulation in diabetes mellitus. Arch Ophthalmol 1986; 104:991–996.
16. Sinclair SH. Macular retinal capillary hemodynamics in diabetic patients. Ophthalmology 1991; 98:1580–1586.
17. Sinclair SH, Grunwald JE, Riva CE, et al. Retinal vascular autoregulation in diabetes mellitus. Ophthalmology 1982; 89:748–750.
18. Ashton N. The pathology of retinal microaneurysms. Acta XVI Concilium Ophthalmol 1950; 1:411–421.
19. Bresnick GH. Background diabetic retinopathy. In: Ryan S, ed. Retina. vol 2. St. Louis: CV Mosby Co; 1990: 327–366.
20. Bloodworth JMB. Diabetic retinopathy. Diabetes 1962; 11:1–22.
21. Benson WE, Brown GC, Tasman W. Diabetes and its ocular complications. Philadelphia: WB Saunders Co; 1988.
22. Kohner EM, Sleightholm M, Kroc Collaborative Study Group. Does microaneurysm count reflect severity of early diabetic retinopathy? Ophthalmology 1986; 93:586–589.
23. Early Treatment Diabetic Retinopathy Study Group. ETDRS Report No 10: Grading diabetic retinopathy from stereoscopic color fundus photographs—an extension of the modified Airlie House classification. Ophthalmology 1991; 98:786–806.
24. Bresnick GH, Condit R, Syrjala S, Palta M, Groo A, Korth K. Abnormalities of the foveal avascular zone in diabetic retinopathy. Arch Ophthalmol 1984; 102:1286–1293.
25. Sleightholm MA, Arnold J, Kohner EM. Diabetic retinopathy: I. The measurement of intercapillary area in normal retinal angiograms. J Diabetic Complications 1988; 11:113–116.
26. Catalano RA, Tanenbaum HL, Majerovics A, et al. White-centered hemorrhages in diabetic retinopathy. Ophthalmology 1987; 94:388–392.
27. Bresnick GH, Davis MD, Myers FL, et al. Clinicopathologic correlations in diabetic retinopathy. II. Clinical and histologic appearances of retinal capillary microaneurysms. Arch Ophthalmol 1977; 95: 1215–1220.
28. Bresnick GH. Diabetic maculopathy: a critical review highlighting diffuse macular edema. Ophthalmology 1983; 90:1301–1317.
29. Bresnick GH. Diabetic macular edema: a review. Ophthalmology 1986; 93:989–997.
30. Early Treatment Diabetic Retinopathy Study Group. ETDRS Report No 1: Photocoagulation for diabetic macular edema. Arch Ophthalmol 1985; 103:1796–1806.
31. Dobree JH. Simple diabetic retinopathy. Evolution of the lesions and therapeutic considerations. Br J Ophthalmol 1970; 54:1–10.
32. Sigurdsson R, Begg IS. Organised macular plaques in exudative diabetic maculopathy. Br J Ophthalmol 1980; 64:392–397.
33. Patz A, Schatz H, Berkow JE, et al. Macular edema: an overlooked complication of diabetic retinopathy. Trans Am Acad Ophthalmol Otolaryngol 1973; 77:34.
34. Tso MOM, Cunha-Vaz JGF, Shin CY, et al. A clinicopathologic study of blood–retinal barrier in experimental diabetes. Invest Ophthalmol Vis Sci 1979; 18 (suppl): 169.
35. Early Treatment Diabetic Retinopathy Study Group. ETDRS Report No 7: Early treatment diabetic retinopathy study design and baseline patient characteristics. Ophthalmology 1991; 98:741–756.
36. Early Treatment Diabetic Retinopathy Study Group. ETDRS Report No 9: Early photocoagulation for diabetic retinopathy. Ophthalmology 1991; 98:766–785.

37. Early Treatment Diabetic Retinopathy Study Group. ETDRS Report No 11: Classification of diabetic retinopathy from fluorescein angiograms. Ophthalmology 1991; 98:807–822.

38. Early Treatment Diabetic Retinopathy Study Group. ETDRS Report No 12: Fundus photographic risk factors for progression of diabetic retinopathy. Ophthalmology 1991; 98:823–833.

39. Sleightholm MA, Aldington SJ, Arnold J, Kohner EM. Diabetic retinopathy: II. Assessment of severity and progression from fluorescein angiograms. J Diabetic Complications 1988; 2:117–120.

40. Klein BEK, Davis MD, Segal P, Long JA, Harris WA, Haug GA, Magli YL, Syrjala S. Diabetic retinopathy. Assessment of severity and progression. Ophthalmology 1984; 91:10–17.

41. Kohner EM, Dollery CT, Bulpitt CJ. Cotton-wool spots in diabetic retinopathy. Diabetes 1969; 18:691–704.

42. Goldbaum MH. Retinal depression sign indicating a small retinal infarct. Am J Ophthalmol 1978; 86:45–55.

43. Kroc Collaborative Study Group. Blood glucose control and the evolution of diabetic retinopathy and albuminuria: a preliminary multicenter trial. N Engl J Med 1984; 311:365–372.

44. Dahl-Jorgensen K, Brinchmann-Hansen O, Hanssen KF, et al. Rapid tightening of blood glucose control leads to transient deterioration of retinopathy in insulin-dependent diabetes mellitus: the Oslo study. Br Med J 1985; 290:811–815.

45. Lauritzen T, Frost-Larsen K, Larsen HW, et al. Two-year experience with continuous subcutaneous insulin infusion in relation to retinopathy and neuropathy. Diabetes 1985; 34(suppl 3):74–79.

46. Davis MD, Norton EWD, Myers FL. The Airlie classification of diabetic retinopathy. In: Goldberg MF, Fine SL, eds. Symposium on the treatment of diabetic retinopathy. Washington DC; Public Health Service Publication No. 1840, US Government Printing Office; 1969.

47. Muraoka K, Shimizu K. Intraretinal neovascularization in diabetic retinopathy. Ophthalmology 1984; 93:1440–1446.

48. Shimizu K, Kobayaski Y, Muraoka K. Midperipheral fundus involvement in diabetic retinopathy. Ophthalmology 1981; 88:601–612.

49. Niki T, Muraoka K, Shimizu K. Distribution of capillary nonperfusion in early-stage diabetic retinopathy. Ophthalmology 1984; 91:1431–1439.

50. Davis MD. Proliferative diabetic retinopathy. In: Ryan SJ, ed. Retina, vol 2. St. Louis: CV Mosby Co; 1989:367–402.

51. Frank RN. On the pathogenesis of diabetic retinopathy. Ophthalmology 1991; 98:586–592.

52. Taylor E, Dobree JH. Proliferative diabetic retinopathy: site and size of initial lesions. Br J Ophthalmol 1970; 54:11–18.

53. Diabetic Retinopathy Study Research Group. A modification on the Airlie House classification of diabetic retinopathy. Report No 7. Invest Ophthalmol Vis Sci. 1981; 21(part 2):210–226.

54. Davis MD. Vitreous contraction in proliferative diabetic retinopathy. Arch Ophthalmol 1965; 74:741–751.

55. Michels RG. Proliferative diabetic retinopathy. Pathophysiology of extraretinal complications and principles of vitreous surgery. Retina 1981; 1:1–17.

56. Abrams GW, Williams GA. "En bloc" excision of diabetic membranes. Am J Ophthalmol 1987; 103:302–308.

57. Bresnick GH, Haight B, DeVenecia G. Retinal wrinkling and macular heterotopia in diabetic retinopathy. Arch Ophthalmol 1979; 97:1890–1895.

58. Charles S, Flinn CE. The natural history of diabetic extramacular traction retinal detachment. Arch Ophthalmol 1981; 99:66–68.

59. Dobree JH. Proliferative diabetic retinopathy: evolution of the retinal lesions. Br J Ophthalmol 1964; 48:637–649.

60. Ramsay WJ, Ramsay RC, Purple RL, Knobloch WH. Involutional diabetic retinopathy. Am J Ophthalmol 1977; 84:851–858.

Diabetic Retinopathy: Practical Management, by R. Joseph Olk and Carol M. Lee. J.B. Lippincott Company, Philadelphia © 1993.

CHAPTER · 3

Review of National Collaborative Studies

DIABETIC RETINOPATHY STUDY

Laser photocoagulation for the treatment of proliferative diabetic retinopathy (PDR) was described in the early 1960s by Meyer-Schwickerath with xenon arc.[1,2] Surface neovascularization was directly treated, and it appeared to regress, probably by direct impediment of the blood flow to the vessels. Laser treatment performed with the ruby laser and, later, with the argon laser, used an indirect scatter pattern, in addition to the direct method of treatment. In the late 1960s, studies noting the regression of the neovascular tissue following laser treatment appeared,[3–5] and the efficacy of laser photocoagulation was tested in several clinical-trials. Two large randomized clinical trials were The British Multicentre Trial using xenon arc[6] and the Diabetic Retinopathy Study (DRS)[7–10] sponsored by the National Eye Institute, using both xenon arc and argon blue-green laser photocoagulation. The latter study demonstrated the efficacy of photocoagulation in the management of proliferative diabetic retinopathy and will be discussed in the next several sections.

The DRS, a multicenter national prospective collaborative effort begun in 1971, was de-signed to answer the question of whether photocoagulation could prevent the development of severe visual loss in eyes with proliferative diabetic retinopathy. With use of both xenon arc and argon blue-green laser, the benefit of laser photocoagulation in the management of certain categories of retinopathy was identified. Retinopathy was classified according to the modified version of the Airlie House Classification[11] of diabetic retinopathy. The original Airlie House scheme refers to a symposium held in 1968 wherein the most current knowledge at that time concerning the natural history and management of diabetic retinopathy was discussed.[12]

Patients who were enrolled in the DRS had proliferative diabetic retinopathy in at least one eye or severe nonproliferative diabetic retinopathy (NPDR) in both eyes, with visual acuity of at least 20/100 in both eyes. *Severe nonproliferative diabetic retinopathy* was defined by the DRS as (1) retinal changes consisting of cotton-wool spots, venous beading, and intra-retinal microvascular abnormalities in at least two of four contiguous overlapping photographic fields; or (2) two of the three findings and moderately severe hemorrhages; and/or microaneurysms in at least one standard photo-

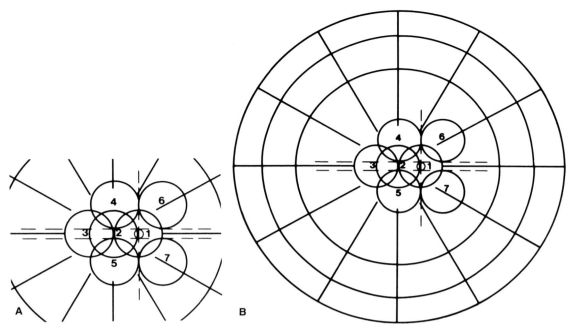

Figure 3–1   Seven standard fields of the modified Airlie House Classification shown for the right eye. Field 1 is centered on the optic disc, field 2 on the macular. Fields 4 to 7 are tangential to horizontal lines passing through the upper and lower poles of the disc and to a vertical line passing through its center. (From DRS No 7. A modification of the Airlie House Classification of diabetic retinopathy. Invest Ophthalmol Vis Sci 1981:21(1); 210–226.)

graphic field.[10] The standard photographic fields are shown in Figure 3-1. One eye of each patient was randomized to treatment with either xenon arc or argon laser photocoagulation and the other to control without treatment. Both treatment techniques included scatter panretinal photocoagulation extending to or beyond the vortex vein ampullae or equator of the eye and focal treatment to surface neovascularization elsewhere (NVE). At first, argon laser was also delivered to elevated NVE and to neovascularization of the disc (NVD) whether on or within one disc diameter of the optic disc, but after a protocol change in 1976, this was no longer required nor used.[13]

Between 1972 and 1975, 1758 patients were enrolled in the DRS. The findings were so overwhelmingly in favor of a treatment benefit that a protocol change was instituted in 1976 to allow the photocoagulation treatment of eyes that had originally been randomized to the control group, and to allow several technical changes, including the preference for argon photocoagulation.[13]

The DRS asked three questions:

1. Does photocoagulation help prevent severe vision loss from proliferative diabetic retinopathy? (Severe visual loss is defined here as visual acuity of less than

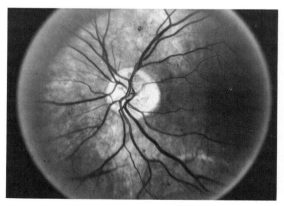

Figure 3–2   Standard photograph 10A. This is the standard against which NVD is compared to determine severity. (From DRS Report 14. Indications for photocoagulation treatment of diabetic retinopathy. Int Opthalmol Clin 1987;27:239–253.)

5/200 at each of two consecutively completed follow-up visits at 4-month intervals.)

2. Is there a difference in the efficacy and safety of extensive scatter and focal treatment to surface NVE, elevated NVE, and NVD with argon laser, and extensive scatter and focal treatment to surface NVE with xenon arc?

3. Which stages of retinopathy benefit most by treatment, and for which stages might treatment be of no benefit or harmful?

The DRS identified four new vessel–vitreous hemorrhage (NV–VH) risk factors or retinopathy risk factors. These were based on (1) the *presence* of new vessels; (2) the *location* of new vessels on or within one disc diameter of the optic disc (NVD); (3) the *severity* of new vessels defined for NVD as equal or greater than standard photograph 10A[11] (Fig. 3-2) or greater than one-fourth to one-third disc area in extent, or for NVE, NVE equal or greater than one-half disc area; and (4) vitreous or preretinal *hemorrhage*. Eyes with three or four retinopathy risk factors were considered to be at highest risk for the development of severe visual loss. When counting risk factors, severity applies to the NVD if both NVD and NVE are present, as it was found that the presence of

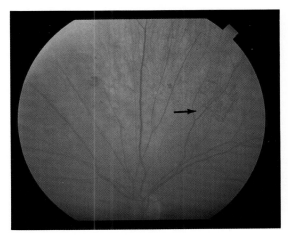

Figure 3–4 An example of two risk factors: NVE greater than one-half disc area (*arrow*), but no other evidence of proliferative disease.

moderate-to-severe NVE when NVD was already present did not contribute to a greater risk of developing severe visual loss[9] (Figs. 3-3, 3-4, 3-5, and 3-6). Three clinical groups were thus identified as being high risk: (1) eyes with NVD greater than or equal to one-fourth to one-third disc diameter in extent (Figs. 3-7 and 3-8); (2) milder NVD if associated with vitreous or preretinal hemorrhage (Figs. 3-9 and 3-10); (3) NVE greater than or equal to one-

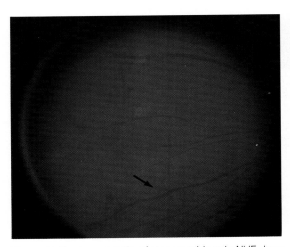

Figure 3–3 An example of an eye with only NVE, less than one-half disc area, and considered to have one risk factor (*arrow*). Note the severe nonproliferative changes and venous beading, in addition to the early proliferative disease. There are also intraretinal blot hemorrhages.

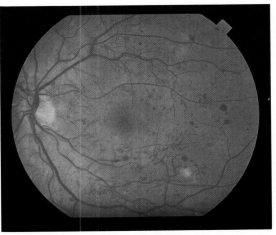

Figure 3–5 An example of high-risk retinopathy with three risk factors: NVD greater than standard photograph 10A, as well as NVE greater than one-half disc area. Here, since there is both NVD and NVE present, the severity of neovascularization refers to the NVD, according to the DRS protocol.

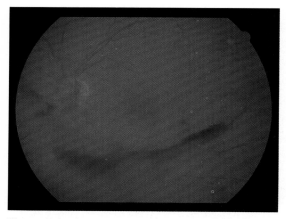

Figure 3–6 An example of a high-risk retinopathy with four risk factors: NVD greater than standard photograph 10A, and preretinal and vitreous hemorrhage.

half disc area in extent if associated with vitreous or preretinal hemorrhage (Figs. 3-11 and 3-12).

After 2 years of follow-up, photocoagulation treatment was found to reduce the risk of severe visual loss by more than 50% in eyes with high-risk retinopathy. At 2 years, 11% of treated eyes and 26% of control eyes with high-risk retinopathy developed severe visual loss; at 4 years, 20% of treated eyes and 44% of control eyes developed severe visual loss. This clear benefit was corroborated in all further reports with longer follow-up[14,15] (Tables 3-1 and 3-2, and Fig. 3-13). A clear treatment benefit, however, was not seen in eyes with early proliferative (less than high-risk retinopathy) or

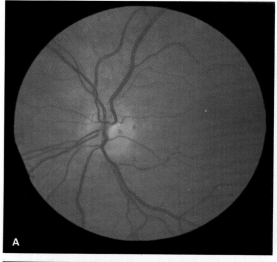

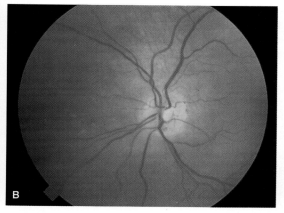

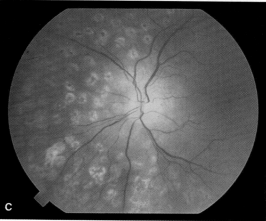

Figure 3–7 (**A**) An example of NVD, less than standard photograph 10A. This 16-year-old white youth with a 15-year history of type I diabetes, was followed every 3 to 4 months with NVD less than 10A. He was followed without any changes over the next year, and (**B**) 1 year after presentation, NVD had increased to the level of standard photograph 10A, with one-fourth to one-third disc diameter of NVD for which the patient received PRP with (**C**) complete resolution of NVD.

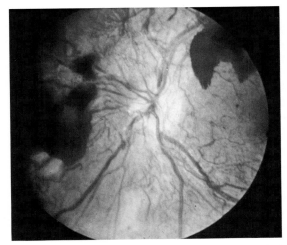

Figure 3–8 An example of severe NVD and preretinal and vitreous hemorrhage with four risk factors: high-risk retinopathy.

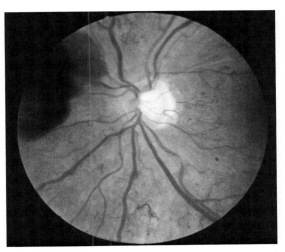

Figure 3–10 An eye with early NVD, early NVE, and preretinal hemorrhage, but high-risk retinopathy. In this patient the severity of vessels relates to the NVD as both NVD and NVE are present.

severe NPDR; because the risk of severe visual loss in these control eyes was small, the DRS did not recommend prompt treatment for these categories of eyes. However, for eyes with high-risk characteristics, the DRS recommended that patients be considered for prompt

photocoagulation treatment (Figs. 3-14 and 3-15).

Side effects of photocoagulation were also studied by the DRS, and a decrease in visual acuity and constriction in peripheral visual field attributed to the treatment occurred more frequently in xenon-treated eyes compared with argon-treated eyes.[13,14] An early persistent decrease in vision was also more common in eyes treated with xenon arc and was attrib-

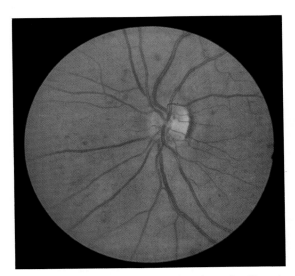

Figure 3–9 An eye with high-risk retinopathy. There is early NVD less than standard photograph 10A, and preretinal hemorrhage along the inferotemporal arcade not seen in this photograph. In counting risk factors for this eye, the NVD is mild (less than standard photograph 10A) and counts for two risk factors plus an additional risk factor for the preretinal hemorrhage, such that this patient has a total of three risk factors.

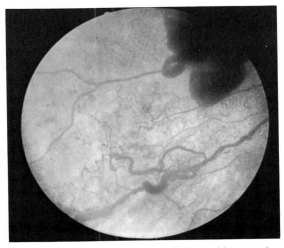

Figure 3–11 An eye with no NVD, but with extensive NVE associated with preretinal hemorrhage. Note, in addition, the significant venous dilation and beading.

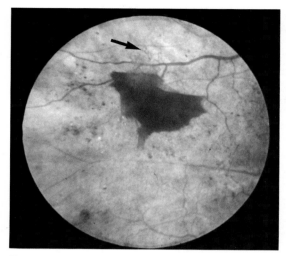

Figure 3–12 An example of high-risk retinopathy, with three risk factors. Note the severe NVE along the infero-temporal vein (*arrow*) and the preretinal hemorrhage just below the NVE.

uted, in part, to increased vitreoretinal traction at the macula owing to contraction of fibro-vascular proliferation.[16] An early transient decrease in visual acuity was also seen more commonly in xenon-treated eyes than in argon-treated eyes and was attributed to an exacerbation of macular edema, if present at the time of initial scatter photocoagulation.[17]

Although the 2-year and 4-year beneficial effects of reducing the incidence of severe visual loss with both xenon- and argon-treated eyes far outweighed the harmful effect of either treatment modality, currently, argon or krypton laser treatment is usually applied in photocoagulation treatment,[13] given the greater side effects of xenon arc. The DRS did not provide a clear recommendation in eyes with less severe proliferative disease or severe NPDR. The Early Treatment Diabetic Retinop-

TABLE 3–1
Cumulative 2-Year Rates of Severe Visual Loss in Eyes Grouped by Baseline Severity of Retinopathy and Treatment Assignment

Retinopathy Severity Group	NVE	NVD	VH/ PRH	No. of NV-VH Risk Factors	Control SVL (%)	Control No. at Risk*	Treated SVL (%)	Treated No. at Risk*	z Value
A	0	0	0	0	3.6	195	3.0	182	0.4
B	0	0	+	1	4.2	11	0.0	16	1.0
C	<½ DA	0	0	1	6.8	120	2.0	96	1.8
D	<½ DA	0	+	2	6.4	18	0.0	19	1.1
E	≥½ DA	0	0	2	6.9	125	4.3	141	1.0
F	≥½ DA	0	+	3	29.7	40	7.2	41	3.0
G	+ or 0	<10A	0	2	10.5	114	3.1	126	2.4
H	+ or 0	<10A	+	3	25.6	39	4.3	35	2.9
I	+ or 0	≥10A	0	3	26.2	150	8.5	174	4.7
J	+ or 0	≥10A	+	4	36.9	76	20.1	107	3.2
All eyes					15.9	897	6.4	946	7.2

NVD, new vessels on or within one disc diameter of the optic disc; NVE, new vessels elsewhere (i.e., outside of the area defined as NVD); VH/PRH, vitreous or preretinal hemorrhage; NV-VH risk factors, new vessels–vitreous hemorrhage risk factors (see text); SVL, severe visual loss (visual acuity < 5/200 at two or more consecutively completed follow-up visits scheduled at 4-month intervals); DA, disc area (NVE < ½ DA indicates that NVE do not equal or exceed one-half the area of the disc in any of the standard photographic fields, NVE ≥ ½ DA indicates that NVE equal or exceed this area in at least one of these fields); 10A, Standard Photograph 10A of the Modified Airlie House Classification.
*In the 20- to 24-month interval.
(From DRS Report No. 14: Indications for photocoagulation treatment of diabetic retinopathy. Int Ophthalmol Clin 1987;27:239–253.)

TABLE 3-2
Cumulative 2- and 4-Year Rates of Severe Visual Loss in Eyes Grouped by Baseline Severity of Retinopathy and Treatment Assignment

Severity of Retinopathy	Table 1 Groups	No. of NV-VH Risk Factors		Control SVL (%)	Control No. at Risk*	Treated SVL (%)	Treated No. at Risk*	z Value
Nonproliferative	A	0	2-yr	3.2	297	2.8	303	0.3
			4-yr	12.8	183	4.3	188	3.6
Proliferative without high-risk characteristics	B–E, G	1 or 2	2-yr	7.0	603	3.2	615	3.1
			4-yr	20.9	332	7.4	390	6.5
Proliferative with high-risk characteristics	F, H–J	3 or 4	2-yr	26.2	473	10.9	570	7.1
			4-yr	44.0	238	20.4	324	8.5
All eyes			2-yr	14.0	1378	6.2	1489	7.4
			4-yr	28.5	754	12.0	903	11.0

NV-VH, new vessel–vitreous hemorrhage risk factors (see text); SVL, severe visual loss (visual acuity < 5/200 at two or more consecutively completed follow-up visits scheduled at 4-month intervals).
*In the 20- to 24-month interval for the 2-year rates and the 44- to 48-month interval for the 4-year rates.
(From DRS Report No. 14: Indications for photocoagulation treatment of diabetic retinopathy. Int Ophthalmol Clin 1987;27:239–253.)

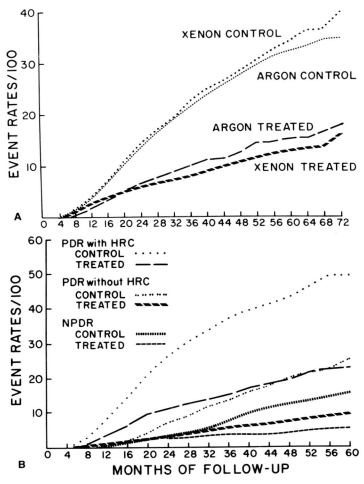

Figure 3-13 (**A**) Cumulative rates of severe visual loss for argon-treated and xenon-treated groups separated. (**B**) Cumulative rates of severe visual loss for eyes classified by the presence of proliferative retinopathy (PDR), high-risk characteristics (HRC), and nonproliferative retinopathy (NPDR) in baseline photographs; argon and xenon groups are combined. (From DRS Report 8. Photocoagulation of proliferative diabetic retinopathy: clinical applications of DRS findings. Ophthalmology 1988; 88:583–600.)

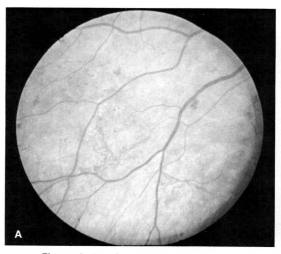
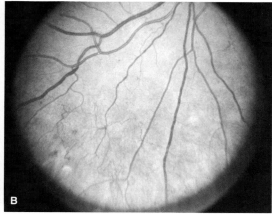

Figure 3–14 An example of two risk factors: Although there is extensive NVE, no NVD or hemorrhage was present. This eye does not meet high-risk retinopathy criteria.

athy Study (ETDRS) addressed this topic within its design (Fig. 3-16).

EARLY TREATMENT DIABETIC RETINOPATHY STUDY

The Early Treatment Diabetic Retinopathy Study is a multicenter collaborative prospective clinical trial sponsored by the National Eye Institute. Between 1980 and 1985, it recruited and enrolled over 3700 patients. The ETDRS addressed three questions:

1. Is photocoagulation effective in the treatment of diabetic macular edema?
2. Is aspirin effective in altering the course of retinopathy?
3. When should panretinal photocoagulation be initiated to be most effective in the management of diabetic retinopathy?[18–24]

The first reports showed that focal photocoagulation of "clinically-significant macular edema" substantially reduced the risk of visual loss when compared with untreated controls.[18–21] *Clinically significant macular edema* was defined by the ETDRS as having any of the following characteristics (Figs. 3-17, 3-18, and 3-19):

> thickening of the retina at or within 500 microns of the center of the macula; hard exudates at or within 500 microns of the center of the macula, if associated with thickening of the adjacent retina and not residual hard exudates remaining after the disappearance of retinal thickening; or a zone or zones of retinal thickening of one disc area or larger, any part of which is within one disc diameter of the center of the macula.[18,19]

In one arm of the study, patients with macular edema and mild-to-moderate diabetic retinopathy in one or both eyes were randomized first to immediate photocoagulation or to deferral of treatment (controls). Of those who

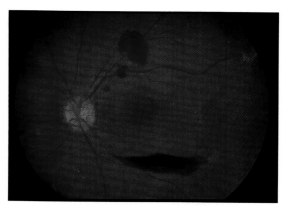

Figure 3–15 An example of high-risk retinopathy with extensive NVD, NVE, preretinal hemorrhage, and fibrovascular proliferation.

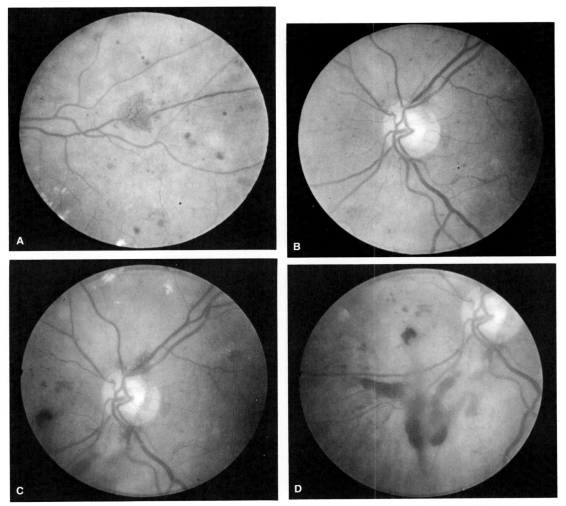

Figure 3–16 (**A**) A patient presented with exudative maculopathy and a small amount of NVE less than one-half disc diameter equivalent to one risk factor retinopathy. Visual acuity was 20/400. (**B**) One year later, she had NVD equal to standard photograph 10A. Although panretinal photocoagulation and grid treatment were recommended for her high-risk retinopathy and macular edema, she refused treatment. (**C–E**) She returned 1 year later with a drop in vision, increased NVD (greater than standard photo 10A), with preretinal and vitreous hemorrhage and diffuse diabetic macular edema. At this point, she consented to treatment. (**F,G**) Fluorescein angiography showed capillary nonperfusion of the posterior pole, leakage of dye from the disc, and blockage from preretinal hemorrhage. (**H**) After completion of her macular and panretinal photocoagulation, 2 years later, she had complete regression of her proliferative disease and no evidence of maculopathy. Visual acuity is 20/100.

(continued)

were immediately treated, further randomization provided them either panretinal photocoagulation, with follow-up focal treatment, or immediate focal treatment only. ETDRS Report No. 1 was based on the comparison between the eyes that received immediate focal photo-coagulation only and those that served as controls with deferral of photocoagulation.

Eyes had to have visual acuity of at least 20/200 and *macular edema,* defined as retinal thickening or definite hard exudates at or within one disc diameter of the center of the

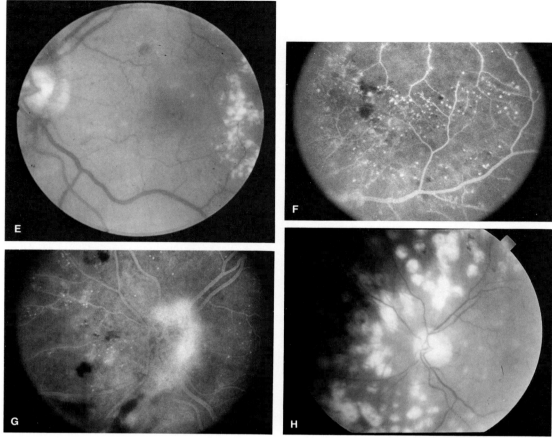

Figure 3–16   (continued)

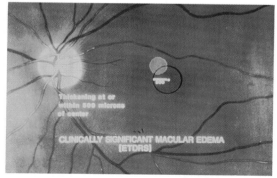

Figure 3–17   Clinically significant macular edema. Retinal thickening at or within 500 μm of the macular center. (From Ferris FL, et al. Photocoagulation for diabetic macular edema: results of the Early Treatment Diabetic Retinopathy Study. Contemp Ophthal Forum 1986; 4:25–31.)

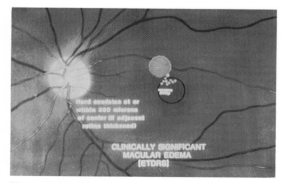

Figure 3–18   Hard exudates at or within 500 μm of the macular center, if associated with thickening of the adjacent retina. (From Ferris FL, et al. Photocoagulation for diabetic macular edema: results of the Early Treatment Retinopathy Study. Contemp Ophthal Forum 1986; 4:25–31.)

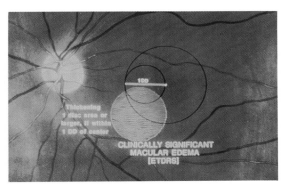

Figure 3–19 Retinal thickening at least one disc area in extent, any part of which is within one disc diameter of the macular center. (From Ferris FL, et al. Photocoagulation for diabetic macular edema: results of the Early Treatment Diabetic Retinopathy Study. Contemp Ophthal Forum 1986; 4:25–31.)

macula.[20] Clinically significant macular edema was further identified by the presence of one or more of the aforementioned characteristics, diagnosed by clinical contact lens biomicroscopy, and documented with stereo fundus photography. Fluorescein angiography was required by the ETDRS only after the clinical determination of "clinically significant macular edema" had been made, to aid in the treatment of angiographically discernible lesions. The definition of macular edema was not fulfilled if only fluorescein leakage was present without clinical retinal thickening. Eyes received focal photocoagulation, including grid photocoagulation in areas of diffuse leakage or capillary nonperfusion within two disc diameters of the center of the macula. Initially, argon blue-green wavelength was used, but later green-only wavelength[18,21] was generally used.

The results showed that focal photocoagulation reduced the risk of visual loss by approximately 50% in eyes with clinically significant macular edema. *Visual loss* was defined here as doubling of the visual angle or a loss of three lines or more on the ETDRS chart. Eyes with clinically significant macular edema affecting the center of the macula showed the greatest benefit with treatment. Eyes with macular edema, but without characteristics meeting clinical significance, did not demonstrate this reduction in visual loss. Finally, eyes with clinically significant characteristics, but without involvement of the center of the macula, showed a beneficial treatment effect midway between the two previously mentioned groups[22] (Fig. 3-20). Almost three-fourths of eyes in this study with clinically significant macular edema had central foveal involvement; at the 1-year and 3-year follow-up visits, central foveal thickening was noted in 50% more eyes randomized to deferral than to treatment. Thus, early focal treatment was also significantly associated with a decrease in the occurrence of retinal thickening involving the center of the macula.

The beneficial effect of this treatment proved greatest in eyes with initially poorer entry visual acuity (worse than 20/40) (Fig. 3-21), but all eyes, despite entry visual acuity, demonstrated this favorable effect. Although visual loss was significantly reduced, visual gain was minimal; thus, the goal of treatment is to "maintain" visual acuity and to prevent worsening of visual acuity caused by untreated macular edema, especially if clinical stereo-biomicroscopic examination confirms that the center of the macula is involved. In such cases, the ETDRS recommends the consideration of prompt treatment, regardless of the visual acuity, since the probability of visual loss without treatment is high.

Recently, the ETDRS reported its findings concerning the second two questions in its design.[23] It found that daily ingestion of 650 mg of aspirin had no demonstrable effects on the progression of diabetic retinopathy in up to 8 years of follow-up.[24] In this trial, 3711 patients with mild-to-severe nonproliferative or early proliferative retinopathy were randomized to daily ingestion of either 650 mg of aspirin or placebo. No significant difference was seen in the development of high-risk retinopathy, in the risk of visual loss, or in the risk of vitreous hemorrhage between eyes of patients receiving aspirin or those receiving placebo, despite randomization to either immediate treatment or to deferral of treatment. Although one study showed an increase in the number of microaneurysms[25] in the eyes of patients receiving placebo (vs aspirin) with mild-to-moderate diabetic retinopathy, neither that study nor the ETDRS could demonstrate any effect on the overall course or progression of retinopathy.

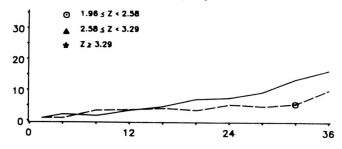

Macular Edema— Not Clinically Significant

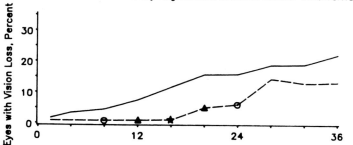

Macular Edema—Clinically Significant without Center Involvement

Figure 3–20 Comparison of percentages of eyes that experienced visual loss of 15 or more letters (equivalent to at least doubling of the initial visual angle) in eyes classified by severity of macular edema in baseline fundic photographs and assigned to either immediate photocoagulation for macular edema (*broken line*) or deferral of photocoagulation unless high-risk characteristics developed (*solid line*). (From ETDRS Report No 4. Photocoagulation for retinal macular edema. Int Ophthalmol Clin 1987; 27:265–272.)

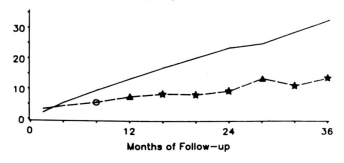

Macular Edema—Clinically Significant with Center Involvement

The ETDRS felt that their findings suggested there was no ophthalmologic contraindication to aspirin use when needed for other medical reasons in patients with mild-to-severe NPDR or early proliferative retinopathy.

The question of when to initiate photocoagulation in the management of diabetic retinopathy is addressed in the recent ninth report of the ETDRS.[26] In this design, 3711 patients with bilateral mild-to-severe nonproliferative or early proliferative (less than high-risk) retinopathy were enrolled. The eyes of patients were divided among those with no macular edema (Fig. 3-22), those with macular edema and less severe retinopathy (Fig. 3-23), and

those with macular edema and more severe retinopathy (Fig. 3-24). One eye of each patient was randomized to deferral of treatment, and one eye of each patient was randomized to early photocoagulation in one of the four treatment strategies of different combinations of panretinal scatter and macular focal photocoagulation, depending on the presence of macular edema and level of retinopathy.

The definitions of terms commonly used in the ETDRS reports are listed in Table 3-3. As seen in the table, mild, moderate, severe, and very severe nonproliferative retinopathy are used to describe those clinical changes referred to historically as background and pre-

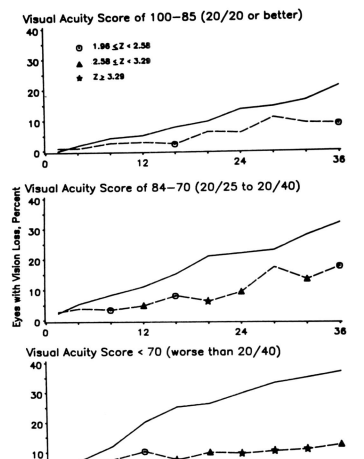

Figure 3–21 Comparison of percentages of eyes that experienced visual loss of 15 or more letters (equivalent to at least a doubling of the visual angle) in eyes with clinically significant macular edema in baseline fundus photographs classified by baseline visual acuity score and assigned to either immediate photocoagulation for macular edema (*broken line*) or deferral of photocoagulation unless high-risk characteristics developed (*solid line*). (From ETDRS Report No 4. Photocoagulation for diabetic macular edema. Int Ophthalmol Clin 1987; 27:265–272.)

proliferative change. We now refer to all retinal changes less than proliferative retinopathy as nonproliferative retinopathy.

Results of this study show that the strategies of photocoagulation involving immediate full scatter reduce the rate of progression to high-risk retinopathy by 50%, whereas those strategies involving immediate mild scatter reduce the rate by 25%. The overall risk of severe visual loss, however, was low for all eyes; even with deferral of treatment, eyes with more severe retinopathy and macular edema experienced only a 6.5% rate of severe visual loss at 5 years. No significant difference was noted in the rate of moderate or severe visual loss in eyes without macular edema between either treatment strategy or deferral of treatment. Early photocoagulation produced a lower rate of severe visual loss at 5 years in eyes with macular edema and less severe retinopathy; but again, the risk was low in all groups, including the deferral group. Although the risk of severe visual loss was reduced from 6.5% at 5 years in eyes with macular edema and more severe retinopathy randomized to deferral to between 3.8% and 4.7% in eyes that received early photocoagulation, this difference was not statistically significant.

Early photocoagulation appeared to have a higher earlier rate of moderate visual loss until

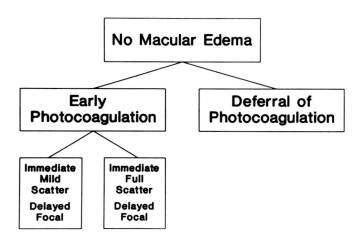

Figure 3–22 Early Treatment Diabetic Retinopathy Study photocoagulation treatment scheme for eyes without macular edema with moderate-to-severe nonproliferative or early proliferative retinopathy. Patients' eyes were assigned randomly to early photocoagulation or deferral of photocoagulation. The eyes assigned to early photocoagulation were further assigned randomly to either mild or full scatter (panretinal) photocoagulation. (From ETDRS Report No 7. Early Treatment Diabetic Retinopathy Study design and baseline characteristics. Ophthalmology 1991; 98:741–756.)

the first year; thereafter, all strategies of early photocoagulation had a lower risk of moderate visual loss. Both the side effect of moderate visual loss and constriction of peripheral visual field appeared to be due to the scatter treatment. These losses were greater in the full-scatter group when compared with the mild-scatter group. The benefit of early reduction in the rate of moderate visual loss in eyes with macular edema appears to be due to the effects of early focal photocoagulation.

The results from this study also showed that early photocoagulation reduces the risk of the need for vitrectomy and the risk of progression to high-risk retinopathy. ETDRS Report No. 9 again reiterated the beneficial effect of focal

photocoagulation on reducing the risk of moderate visual loss in eyes with clinically significant macular edema.[26]

The ETDRS also studied the rate of progression from nonproliferative and early proliferative disease to the high-risk stages.[26,27] They identified certain characteristics within the level of severe NPDR that tended to have a higher risk of progression to high-risk retinopathy; this will be discussed in more detail in Chapter 4. Eyes with baseline, severe nonproliferative diabetic retinopathy developed high-risk retinopathy at a rate of 17% by 1 year of follow-up, 44% by 3 years of follow-up, and 58% by 5 years of follow-up. In eyes with intraretinal characteristics consistent with se-

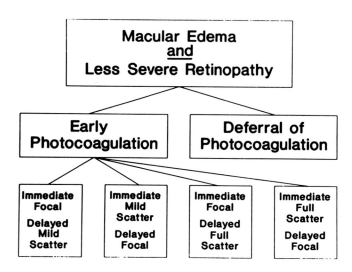

Figure 3–23 Early Treatment Diabetic Retinopathy Study photocoagulation treatment scheme for eyes with macular edema and *less severe retinopathy* (mild-to-moderate nonproliferative retinopathy). Eyes were assigned randomly to early photocoagulation or to deferral of photocoagulation. Eyes assigned to early photocoagulation were further assigned randomly to either mild or full scatter (panretinal) photocoagulation, and to either immediate focal or delayed focal treatment. In eyes assigned to immediate focal treatment, the assigned scatter treatment was not applied initially, but only if severe nonproliferative retinopathy or worse developed during follow-up. (From ETDRS Report No 7. Early Treatment Diabetic Retinopathy Study design and baseline patient characteristics. Ophththalmology 1991; 98:741–756.)

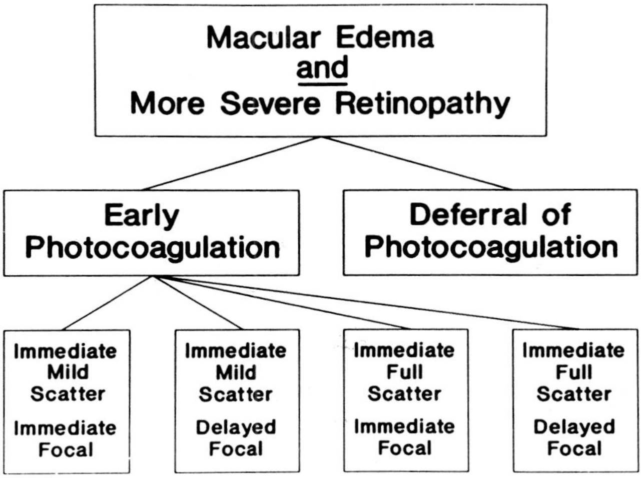

Figure 3–24 Early Treatment Diabetic Retinopathy Study photocoagulation treatment scheme for eyes with macular edema and *more severe retinopathy*. The patients' eyes were assigned randomly to immediate photocoagulation or to deferral of photocoagulation. Eyes assigned to immediate photocoagulation were further assigned randomly to either mild or full scatter (panretinal) photocoagulation, and to either immediate focal treatment or to delayed focal treatment for at least 4 months. (From ETDRS Report No 7. Early Treatment Diabetic Retinopathy Study design and baseline patient characteristics. Ophthalmology 1991; 98:741–746.)

TABLE 3–3
Definitions of Commonly Used Terms

A. **Macular edema**

Thickening of retina within one disc diameter of the center of the macula; or hard exudates $\geq$ standard photograph 3 in a standard 30° photographic field centered on the macula (field 2), with some hard exudates within one disc diameter of the center of the macula

B. **Clinically significant macular edema (CSME)**

Retinal thickening at or within 500 μm of the center of the macula; or hard exudates at or within 500 μm of the center of the macula, if associated with thickening of the adjacent retina; or a zone or zones of retinal thickening one disc area in size at least part of which was within one disc diameter of the center.

C. **Mild nonproliferative retinopathy**

At least one microaneurysm; and definition not met for D, E, F, or G below

D. **Moderate nonproliferative retinopathy**

Hemorrhages or microaneurysms $\geq$ standard photograph 2A; and/or soft exudates, venous beading, or intraretinal microvascular abnormalities definitely present; and definition not met for E, F, or G below

E. **Severe nonproliferative retinopathy**

Soft exudates, venous beading, and intraretinal microvascular abnormalities all definitely present in at least two of fields 4 through 7; or two of the preceding three lesions present in at least two of fields 4 through 7 and hemorrhages and microaneurysms present in these four fields, equaling or exceeding standard photo 2A in at least one of them; or intraretinal microvascular abnormalities present in each of fields 4 through 7 and equaling or exceeding standard photograph 8A in at least two of them; and definition not met for F or G below

F. **Early proliferative retinopathy** (i.e., proliferative retinopathy without DRS high-risk characteristics)

New vessels, and definition not met for G below

G. **High-risk proliferative retinopathy** (proliferative retinopathy with DRS high-risk characteristics)

New vessels on or within one disc diameter of the optic disc (NVD) $\geq$ standard photograph 10A (about one-fourth to one-third disc area), with or without vitreous or preretinal hemorrhage; or vitreous or preretinal hemorrhage accompanied by new vessels, either NVD < standard photograph 10A or new vessels elsewhere (NVE) $\geq$ one-fourth disc area

H. **Less severe retinopathy**

Mild or moderate nonproliferative retinopathy

I. **More severe retinopathy**

Severe nonproliferative or early proliferative retinopathy

J. **Severe visual loss**

Visual acuity < 5/200 at two consecutive follow-up visits (scheduled at 4-month intervals)

K. **Moderate visual loss**

Loss of 15 or more letters between baseline and follow-up visit, equivalent to a doubling of the initial visual angle (i.e., 20/20 to 20/40 or 20/50 to 20/100)

(From ETDRS Report No. 7. Early treatment diabetic retinopathy study design and patient characteristics. Ophthalmology 1991;98:741–756.)

vere nonproliferative diabetic retinopathy, 15% by 1 year, 40% by 3 years, and 56% by 5 years had progressed to the high-risk stage. A subset of severe NPDR eyes, called very severe NPDR, had 45% by 1 year, 65% by 3 years, and 71% by 5 years progress to the high-risk stage.[26]

However, only a small benefit of early photocoagulation was noted because both eyes receiving early treatment and eyes that were deferred had a low rate of severe visual loss. Since over 50% of certain eyes with both less and more severe retinopathy can be expected to develop high-risk characteristics in 3 to 5 years, eyes that are in this category need to be followed carefully. The ETDRS states that scatter photocoagulation can be considered, although it is not necessarily recommended at this stage, given its side effects, such as decreased peripheral visual field and paracentral visual scotomas. If both eyes are reaching the high-risk stage, initiating early photocoagulation in one eye is recommended, and if an eye develops high-risk retinopathy, panretinal photocoagulation should unequivocally be initiated.

DIABETIC RETINOPATHY VITRECTOMY STUDY

Machemer originally described the use of vitrectomy in the management of diabetic non-clearing vitreous hemorrhage of over 1-year duration or in tractional detachment of the center of the macula.[28] The indications and uses of vitrectomy over the last 20 years have changed, and many authors have since discussed the indications and appropriate timing of such surgery.[28-34] The Diabetic Retinopathy Vitrectomy Study (DRVS) was established by the National Eye Institute to address the question of when to perform vitrectomy in the management of severe proliferative disease. Thus, the DRVS studied the natural history of severe proliferative disease and explored the possible benefits and timing of vitrectomy surgery in diabetic eyes.[35-39]

Between 1976 and 1980, the DRVS followed 744 eyes of 622 patients with severe proliferative retinopathy using conventional management, including photocoagulation.[35] Of the eyes followed for their natural course, visual acuity dropped from 10/30 to 10/50 at baseline to less than 5/200 at 2 years in 45% of eyes, if they originally had greater than four disc areas of new vessels.[35] Visual acuity dropped to less than 5/200 in 14% of eyes having baseline extramacular traction detachments without active new vessels or vitreous hemorrhage at entry.[35] Vitrectomy was needed in 25% of these eyes after 2 years of follow-up owing to either new macular detachments or to hemorrhage that did not clear after 1 year of follow-up.[35] The efficacy of vitrectomy performed earlier than 1 year after the occurrence of vitreous hemorrhage was investigated because of the high rate of severe visual loss and high incidence of vitrectomy surgery required during follow-up. At the time when the DRVS was formulated, most surgeons waited for at least 1 year following severe vitreous hemorrhage before performing vitrectomy.

In one strategy, 616 eyes with recent severe vitreous hemorrhage, obscuring at least all of the posterior pole and having visual acuity of less than or equal to 5/200 for at least 1 month, were randomized to early vitrectomy or conventional management with deferral of vitrectomy for at least 1 year.[36] Recovery of good vision, defined as visual acuity of 10/20 or better, was seen in the early vitrectomy group, as was an increased incidence of loss of light perception. The increase in no light perception vision in the early vitrectomy group was statistically significant only up until the 18-month follow-up; thereafter, the difference was not significant.[36,39] Patients were divided by subgroup of diabetes. *Type I* was defined as patients currently receiving insulin whose diabetes was diagnosed at or before age 20. *Type II* was defined as patients whose diabetes was diagnosed at 40 years of age or older, regardless of insulin use, and an intermediate mixed group consisted of patients whose diabetes was diagnosed between ages 21 and 39.

The DRVS found that a clear-cut advantage was seen in early vitrectomy for type I diabetics as compared with eyes in the control group at the 2-year follow-up visit.[36] The early-treatment group maintained a higher proportion of eyes with 10/20 or better at both the 2-year and 4-year follow-up periods, especially for patients with type I diabetes.[39] By 2 years, 36% of type I diabetic eyes undergoing early vitrectomy had recovery of good vision greater than or equal to 10/20, compared with 12% of eyes managed conventionally.[36] By 4 years, 50% of type I diabetic eyes undergoing early vitrectomy had maintained visual acuity of 10/20 or better, compared with 10% managed conventionally.[39] However, in eyes of patients with type II diabetes and in the mixed group, little difference was noted between the two treatment strategies at both the 2-year and 4-year visits.[39] In the deferral group, spontaneous clearing of the vitreous hemorrhage occurred in 29% of type II eyes, 21% of mixed group eyes, and 16% of type I eyes, indicating that deferral of vitrectomy in type II and mixed group eyes may be an acceptable alternative, if the fellow eye had good vision.[39] However, the significant advantage of early vitrectomy is clearly seen for type I diabetic eyes with severe vitreous hemorrhage.

Three hundred seventy eyes with active and advanced proliferative diabetic retinopathy and useful baseline vision, defined as visual acuity of 10/200 or better, were also randomized to early vitrectomy or conventional management.[37] The proportion of eyes with a good visual outcome, defined as visual acuity of 10/20 or better, was higher in the early vitrectomy group at each follow-up visit after the 3-month visit up until the last reported visit at 4 years. This difference was statistically significant at each of the follow-up visits, except the 6-month and 24-month visits.[37] There was no significant difference between eyes undergoing early vitrectomy versus eyes followed by conventional management in the development of severe visual loss or no light perception vision, although more eyes had no light perception vision in follow-up for the early vitrectomy group.[37] In addition, no specific advantages were seen in any of the three subtypes of diabetes. The increased advantage of early vitrectomy was directly correlated with the severity

of vessel abnormalities. The greatest advantage of early vitrectomy over deferral in achieving a good visual outcome was seen in eyes with the worst retinopathy at entry. In each of the studies, eyes randomized to conventional management were eligible for surgery before 1 year if retinal detachment involving the macula occurred.

The DRVS, then, advocated early vitrectomy for eyes with severe visual loss from nonclearing vitreous hemorrhage of at least 1-month duration in type I diabetics and in monocular patients whose fellow eye does not provide useful vision, despite the type of diabetes, bearing in mind the increased incidence of early loss of light perception vision. Early vitrectomy should also be considered in eyes with useful vision and advanced active proliferative retinopathy not as a replacement, but as an adjunct modality of treatment when new vessels have not sufficiently regressed following photocoagulation or if hemorrhage precludes photocoagulation treatment. It should be noted that the DRVS did not employ the endophotocoagulation technique and that the techniques of vitreoretinal surgery are constantly evolving, limiting these findings to only a part of the decision of when to perform vitrectomy in the management of severe proliferative diabetic retinopathy, as will be discussed in Chapter 7.

References

1. Meyer-Schwickerath G. Light coagulation. St Louis: CV Mosby Co; 1960.
2. Meyer-Schwickerath G, Gerke E. Bjerum Lecture: treatment of diabetic retinopathy with photocoagulation. Acta Ophthalmol 1983; 61:756–768.
3. Aiello LM, Beethan WP, Balodimas MC. Ruby laser photocoagulation in treatment of diabetic proliferating retinopathy. In: Goldberg MF, Fine SL, eds. Symposium on the treatment of diabetic retinopathy. Public Health Service Publication No. 1890, Washington, DC: US Government Printing Office; 1969.
4. Okun E. Summary of papers on treatment techniques in photocoagulation. In: Goldberg MF, Fine SL, eds. Symposium on the treatment of diabetic retinopathy. Public Health Service Publication No. 1890, Washington, DC: US Government Printing Office; 1969.
5. Zweng HC. The treatment of diabetic retinopathy by laser photocoagulation. In: Goldberg MF, Fine SL, eds. Symposium on the treatment of diabetic reti-

nopathy. Public Health Service Publication No. 1890, Washington, DC: US Government Printing Office; 1969.

6. British Multicentre Study Group. Photocoagulation for PDR. A randomized trial using xenon arc. Diabetologia 1984; 26:109–115.

7. Diabetic Retinopathy Study Research Group. Preliminary report on effects of photocoagulation therapy. Am J Ophthalmol 1976; 81:383–396.

8. Diabetic Retinopathic Study Research Group. Photocoagulation treatment of proliferative diabetic retinopathy: the second report of diabetic retinopathy/vitrectomy study findings. Am J Ophthalmol 1978; 85:82–106.

9. Diabetic Retinopathy Study Research Group. DRS Report No. 3: Four risk factors for severe visual loss in diabetic retinopathy. Arch Ophthalmol 1979; 97:654–655.

10. Diabetic Retinopathy Study Research Group. DRS Report No 6: Design, methods, and baseline results. Invest Ophthalmol Vis Sci 1981; 21:149–209.

11. Diabetic Retinopathy Study Research Group. DRS Report No. 7: A modification on the Airlie House classification of diabetic retinopathy. Invest Ophthalmol Vis Sci 1981; 21(part 2):210–226.

12. Goldberg MF, Jampol LM. Knowledge of diabetic retinopathy before and 18 years after the Airlie House Symposium on treatment of diabetic retinopathy. Ophthalmology 1987; 94:741–746.

13. Diabetic Retinopathy Study Research Group. DRS Report No 8: Photocoagulation treatment of proliferative diabetic retinopathy: clinical applications of DRS findings. Ophthalmology 1981; 88:583–600.

14. Diabetic Retinopathic Study Research Group. DRS Report No 4: Diabetes 1979. International Congress Series No. 500. Proceedings of the 10th Congress of the Internal Diabetes Federation, Vienna, Austria, September 1979; 789–794.

15. Diabetic Retinopathy Study Research Group. DRS Report No 14: Indications for photocoagulation treatment of diabetic retinopathy. Int Ophthalmol Clin 1987; 274:239–252.

16. Diabetic Retinopathy Study Research Group. DRS Report No 5: Photocoagulation treatment of proliferative diabetic retinopathy: relationship of adverse treatment effects to retinopathy severity. Dev Ophthalmol 1981; 2:248–261.

17. Ferris FL, Podgor MJ, Davis MD, Diabetic Retinopathy Study Research Group. DRS Report No 12: Macular edema in diabetic retinopathy study patients. Ophthalmology 1987; 94:754–760.

18. Early Treatment Diabetic Retinopathy Study Research Group. ETDRS Report No 1: Photocoagulation for diabetic macular edema. Arch Ophthalmol 1985; 103:1796–1806.

19. Ferris FL et al. Photocoagulation for diabetic macular edema: results of the Early Treatment Diabetic Retinopathy Study. Contemp Ophthalmic Forum; 1986; 4:25–31.

20. Early Treatment Diabetic Retinopathy Study Research Group. ETDRS Report No 2: Treatment techniques and clinical guidelines for photocoagulation of diabetic macular edema. Ophthalmology 1987; 94:761–774.

21. Early Treatment Diabetic Retinopathy Study Research Group. ETDRS Report No 3: Techniques for scatter and local photocoagulation treatment of diabetic retinopathy. Int Ophthalmol Clin 1987; 27:254–264.

22. Early Treatment Diabetic Retinopathy Study Research Group. ETDRS Report No 4: Photocoagulation for diabetic macular edema. Int Ophthalmol Clin 1987; 27:265–272.

23. Early Treatment Diabetic Retinopathy Study Research Group. ETDRS Report No 7: Early treatment diabetic retinopathy study design and baseline patient characteristics. Ophthalmology 1991; 98:741–756.

24. Early Treatment Diabetic Retinopathy Study Research Group. ETDRS Report No 8: Effects of aspirin treatment on diabetic retinopathy. Ophthalmology 1991; 98:757–765.

25. DAMAD Study Group. Effect of ASA alone and ASA plus dipyridamole in early diabetic retinopathy. Diabetes 1989; 38:491–498.

26. Early Treatment Diabetic Retinopathy Study Group. ETDRS Report No 9: Early photocoagulation for diabetic retinopathy. Ophthalmology 1991; 98:766–785.

27. Early Treatment Diabetic Retinopathy Study Group. ETDRS Report No 12: Fundus photographic risk factors for progression of diabetic retinopathy. Ophthalmology 1991; 98:823–833.

28. Machemer R, Buettner H, Norton EWD, et al. Vitrectomy: a pars plana approach. Trans Am Acad Ophthalmol Otolaryngol 1971; 75:813–820.

29. Machemer R, Blankenship G. Vitrectomy for proliferative diabetic retinopathy associated with vitreous hemorrhage. Ophthalmology 1981; 88:643–646.

30. Shea M. Early vitrectomy in proliferative diabetic retinopathy. Arch Ophthalmol 1983; 101:1204–1205.

31. Michels RG, Rice TA, Rice EF. Vitrectomy for diabetic vitreous hemorrhage. Am J Ophthalmol 1983; 95:12–21.

32. O'Hanley GP, Canny CLB. Diabetic dense premacular hemorrhage. Ophthalmology 1985; 92:507–511.

33. Ramsay RC, Knoblock WH, Cantrill HL. Timing of vitrectomy for active proliferative diabetic retinopathy. Ophthalmology 1986; 93:283–289.

34. Aaberg TM, Abrams GW. Changing indications and techniques for vitrectomy in management of complications of diabetic retinopathy. Ophthalmology 1987; 94:775–779.

35. Diabetic Retinopathy Vitrectomy Study Group. DRVS Report No 1: Two-year course of visual acuity in severe proliferative diabetic retinopathy with conventional management. Ophthalmology 1985; 92:492–502.

36. Diabetic Retinopathy Vitrectomy Study Group. DRVS Report No 2: Early vitrectomy for severe vitreous hemorrhage in diabetic retinopathy. Two-year results of a randomized trial. Arch Ophthalmol 1985; 103:1644–1652.

37. Diabetic Retinopathy Vitrectomy Study Group. DRVS Report No 3: Early vitrectomy for severe proliferative diabetic retinopathy in eyes with useful vision. Results of a randomized trial. Ophthalmology 1988; 95:1307–1320.

38. Diabetic Retinopathy Vitrectomy Study Group. DRVS Report No 4: Early vitrectomy for severe proliferative diabetic retinopathy in eyes with useful vision. Clinical application of results of a randomized trial. Ophthalmology 1988; 95:1321–1334.

39. Diabetic Retinopathy Vitrectomy Study Group. DRVS Report No 5: Early vitrectomy for severe vitreous hemorrhage in diabetic retinopathy. Four-year results of a randomized trial. Arch Ophthalmol 1990; 108:958–964.

CHAPTER · 4

Management of Nonproliferative Diabetic Retinopathy

All diabetic patients need a dilated fundus examination by an ophthalmologist or specifically trained ophthalmoscopist. The recently published *Preferred Practice Pattern* of the American Academy of Ophthalmology on the evaluation and management of diabetic retinopathy offers a useful guideline.[1] Our guidelines are based on both the natural history of the disease and the individual circumstances in which the clinical findings present.

The Early Treatment Diabetic Retinopathy Study (ETDRS) recently published a clinically useful grading system to identify eyes at a higher risk for developing proliferative and, more importantly, high-risk retinopathy.[2–5] The division of retinopathy into nonproliferative and proliferative, and the further subdivision of the former category into mild, moderate, severe, and very severe does exactly that. *Mild* nonproliferative retinopathy consists of at least one microaneurysm or intraretinal hemorrhage.[2,4] Hard and soft exudates may or may not be present. *Moderate* nonproliferative retinopathy includes eyes with moderate microaneurysms or intraretinal hemorrhages or early mild intraretinal microvascular abnor-

malities (IRMA). Hard or soft exudates may be present.[2,4]

Eyes with mild nonproliferative retinopathy have a low rate of progression to high-risk proliferative disease in 1 year.[4,5] Only 1% will develop high-risk retinopathy in 1 year; but by 5 years, 15% will develop high-risk retinopathy.[4]

Eyes with moderate nonproliferative retinopathy also have a reasonably low rate of progression to proliferative disease within 1 year.[4] Only 3% will develop high-risk disease within 1 year; but by 5 years, 27% will develop high-risk disease.[4]

In contrast, the ETDRS has identified eyes with a much higher rate of progression to neovascular disease (i.e., severe nonproliferative retinopathy). Three characteristics have been shown to individually and collectively herald this higher rate of progression and are represented by the *4-2-1 rule* as presented by Davis, Murphy, and others of the ETDRS.[5] Any one of the following three characteristics constitutes *severe* nonproliferative diabetic retinopathy:

- Four quadrants of severe microaneurysms or intraretinal hemorrhages
- Two quadrants of venous beading

- One quadrant of at least moderately severe IRMA.[5]

Very severe nonproliferative disease is defined by an eye having any two of the three characteristics in the 4-2-1 rule.[5] These eyes have a particularly high rate of advancement to proliferative disease. Of eyes with severe NPDR, 15% developed high-risk retinopathy by 1 year; by 5 years, 56% developed high-risk disease.[4] Of eyes with very severe NPDR, 45% developed high-risk disease after 1 year. By 5 years, 71% had developed high-risk disease.[4,5] Thus, the 4-2-1 rule is a useful clinical measure in predicting the chances that an eye will rapidly progress to proliferative disease.[5]

MANAGEMENT OF MILD-TO-MODERATE NONPROLIFERATIVE DIABETIC RETINOPATHY

The clinical findings of mild-to-moderate NPDR, as stated in Chapter 2, include microaneurysms, dot-and-blot and flame-shaped intraretinal hemorrhages, hard exudates, and macular edema. All of these findings should be visible on the dilated fundus examination. Many studies have evaluated the efficiency and ability of health care professionals to detect diabetic eye disease by ophthalmoscopy,[6–11] especially as related to the efficiency of detecting retinopathy by fundus photography. The correlation between the two techniques is high, especially in eyes with more severe retinopathy, such as neovascularization of the disc (NVD) or elsewhere (NVE).

The less severe forms of retinopathy, such as microaneurysms alone, can be missed by just the clinical examination without the documentation by fundus photography, as seen in one study by Moss and associates, who used direct or indirect ophthalmoscopy.[6] However, overall agreement was quite high, at 86%, between the ophthalmoscopic and photographic gradings for retinopathy. Only one of 1949 eyes reviewed in this study had high-risk retinopathy that was missed on the clinical examination,

whereas retinopathy that is "undercalled" or missed by a clinical examiner is almost always one of less severity.[6,7] Another study by Palmberg and colleagues found that photography was twice as sensitive in detecting early retinopathy, when compared with detection by direct ophthalmoscopy alone.[8] Overall, dilated fundus examination with both direct and indirect ophthalmoscopy is reported to be between 79% and 96% sensitive relative to the use of photography in detecting proliferative disease[6,7] and at least 93% specific in detecting proliferative disease. These figures are based on the assumption that fundus photography can detect 100% of retinopathy. This, of course, is dependent on the individual grader who reviews the photographs.

Guidelines for Follow-Up

Both the natural history of diabetic retinopathy and our ability to detect early retinopathy dictate a scheme for follow-up of a patient with diabetes. Several epidemiologic studies have looked at the progression from early to advanced retinopathy.[7,15] The prevalence of retinopathy increases directly with duration of disease, as seen in the Wisconsin Epidemiologic Study of Diabetic Retinopathy (WESDR) and other reports.[12–20] In patients with diabetes that is diagnosed at younger than 30 years of age, the WESDR found that 59% of persons who had no retinopathy at baseline had some retinopathy by 4 years, and that 41% of eyes with any retinopathy at baseline showed progression of their retinopathy by 4 years.[18] Of those without any retinopathy at baseline, only 1, or 0.4%, of 160 persons who developed retinopathy developed proliferative disease by the 4-year visit.[18] Of those persons with less than proliferative retinopathy at baseline, 41% showed progression of their retinopathy, 4% improved, and 55% demonstrated no change from their baseline examination.[18] Of those showing progression, 26% progressed to proliferative disease.[18]

In persons whose diabetes is diagnosed at age 30 years or older, the WESDR found that 47% of insulin users who were free of retinopathy at baseline developed some retinopathy by 4 years, and 34% developed progression of their disease if they had any retinopathy at baseline examination.[19] Of those with no retinopathy at baseline, none of the insulin users developed proliferative disease. Of persons with less than proliferative retinopathy at baseline, 34% developed progression of their disease, 8% improved, and 58% demonstrated no change at their 4-year examination. Of those with progression of their retinopathy, 22% progressed to proliferative disease.[19]

In eyes of non–insulin-dependent patients with a diagnosis of diabetes at 30 years of age or older, 34% with no retinopathy at baseline had developed some retinopathy at the 4-year visit.[19] Only two persons (0.4%) developed proliferative disease after 4 years from a baseline examination free of retinopathy. Of those with less than proliferative retinopathy at baseline, 25% developed progression of their disease. Of those with progression of their retinopathy, 9% developed proliferative disease at 4 years.[19]

Multiple screening strategies have been employed in cost-effectiveness models in the care and management of diabetic retinopathy[1,9–11] to decrease the incidence of complications, such as visual loss owing to untreated or undetected proliferative disease. The expected progression from no retinopathy to proliferative disease is low in the first several years after diagnosis in juvenile-onset diabetes, although the natural history of the disease grows progressively worse with increasing duration.[15,16] The development of proliferative disease is seen after a shorter duration of diabetes in older-onset diabetics,[13,15,16,19,20] reflecting the difficulty in precisely determining when older-onset diabetes occurs, and increases dramatically after a short lag time relative to duration in both older- and younger-onset diabetics.

Considering the cost-effectiveness models relative to the natural history of the disease and the efficacy of timely detection and treatment of diabetic retinopathy, we agree with the American Academy of Ophthalmology's recommended schedule for the first examination (Table 4-1). If the age of onset is up to 30 years, the first examination should take place by 5 years after onset; if the age of onset is 31 years

or older, the first examination should take place at the time of diagnosis. If diabetes is diagnosed during pregnancy, the first examination recommendations should take place during the first trimester. We agree with their recommendation considering that the prevalence of significant disease in younger-onset diabetic patients has been shown to be very low within the first 4 years of diagnosis. However, it is possible that earlier screening may provide earlier initiation of programmed ophthalmologic care, improved follow-up, and enhanced patient awareness of the importance of early detection of diabetic retinopathy.[11]

Patients with very minimal to no retinopathy at their first examination should be reexamined the following year. This should include a fully dilated examination, because the sensitivity of ophthalmoscopy has been reported to decrease by almost 50% if eyes are not dilated.[6,21] Both direct and indirect ophthalmoscopy should be employed for an adequate magnified examination of the retina. The optic disc and posterior pole are readily viewed with the direct ophthalmoscope. A wider field of view is provided by the indirect ophthalmoscope for examining the periphery of the retina. Slit-lamp biomicroscopy, with either a hand-held or contact lens, is needed for stereoscopic examination of the macula to look for retinal thickening. Gonioscopic evaluation of the angle structures is also recommended to aid in the detection of early neovascularization of the angle.

If either minimal or no retinopathy is found and the best corrected visual acuity is consis-

TABLE 4–1
Timing of the First Dilated Ophthalmologic Examination*

Age at Onset of Diabetes	First Examination Performed
0–30	By 5 years after onset
Over 30	When diagnosis is made
While pregnant[†]	During first trimester

*Following American Academy of Ophthalmology Preferred Practice Pattern: Diabetic Retinopathy
[†]Not gestational diabetes

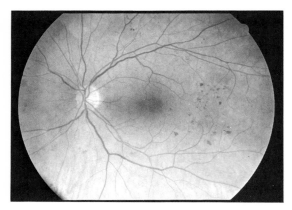

Figure 4–1 An example of mild nonproliferative diabetic retinopathy with microaneurysms and dot-and-blot hemorrhage. There is no evidence of macular edema or proliferative disease at this time. The patient was followed with semiannual examinations. Fundus photographs are useful in this situation to document and compare the progression of the disease. Fluorescein angiography is not indicated.

tent with the clinical findings, fluorescein angiography is not indicated. The role of fundus stereophotography is less clear in these very minimally affected eyes, but can provide documentation for comparison with future findings. In general, in eyes with no retinopathy, no macular edema, or less than mild nonproliferative change, fundus photography is usually unnecessary.

Eyes with mild-to-moderate retinopathy, greater than a rare microaneurysm, but with-

out macular edema, should be reevaluated in 6 months, given that the rate of progression to a more advanced level is higher than the corresponding rate from no retinopathy.[18,19] However, the rate of progression to either any proliferative disease or to high-risk disease at 1 year is low enough to allow semiannual evaluation.[4] Again fluorescein angiography is not indicated, unless there is unexplained visual loss, inconsistent with the clinical findings (Figs. 4-1 and 4-2).

Fundus stereophotographs can be useful in documenting nonproliferative retinopathy and as a permanent library for comparison with future evaluations. We recommend the seven standard photographic fields of the modified Airlie House classification,[22] which have been traditionally used to photograph the retina and document disease[3,6,8,22] (Fig. 4-3). Pairs of fundus stereophotographs enable the examiner to confirm the findings of stereobiomicroscopic examination of the macula. Larger 60° fields are also useful in documenting retinopathy. Color fundus photographs are especially useful when the clinical examination appears to be changing or if the disease appears particularly aggressive, with rapid progression. Photography is also helpful in gauging a response to treatment if photocoagulation is being performed for proliferative disease. If an eye reveals retinopathy that is greater than mild-to-moderate nonproliferative retinopathy or

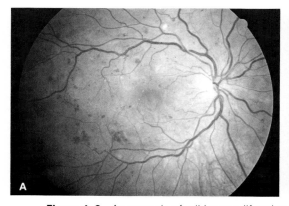
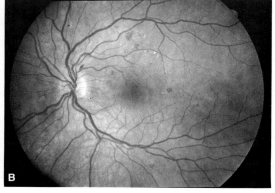

Figure 4–2 An example of mild nonproliferative retinopathy in the left eye and moderate nonproliferative retinopathy in the right eye. (**A**) Microaneurysms, dot-and-blot hemorrhage, minimal exudate, and one cotton-wool spot superiorly are seen in the right eye. (**B**) Hard exudate, dot-and-blot hemorrhages, and one nerve fiber layer hemorrhage just above the optic nerve are seen in the left eye.

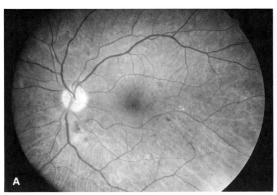

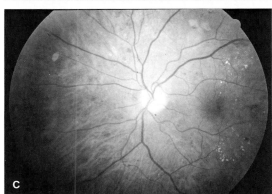

Figure 4–3 (**A**) A 50-year-old man presented with a 2-year history of non-insulin–dependent diabetes and mild nonproliferative diabetic retinopathy. He was followed over the next 7 years without significant change. (**B**) A slight increase in exudate, but no retinal thickening at or within 500 μm of the center of the FAZ is seen. (**C**) This eye remained essentially stable over the next 2 years. Color fundus photographs are helpful to compare and note progression or regression of retinopathy. In the patient's last examination there was a slight increase in his exudate again, but he had no indication for either macular or panretinal treatment.

includes macular thickening, more frequent evaluations will be necessary. This will be discussed in the following sections.

The WESDR recently reported a statistically significant association between the level of serum cholesterol and severity of hard exudates in insulin-using persons, both those with younger- and older-onset disease.[23] We recommend that patients with an overall preponderance of hard exudate at any level of retinopathy have their serum cholesterol levels checked.

In summary (Table 4-2), eyes with no or minimal retinopathy at baseline examination, such as a rare microaneurysm only, may be followed annually. Fundus photography is probably unnecessary, and fluorescein angiography is unnecessary if the visual acuity corresponds to the clinical findings. Eyes with mild-to-moderate nonproliferative retinopathy should be seen at 6-month intervals to look for evolution of their disease. These eyes will benefit

TABLE 4–2
Recommended Follow-Up Schedule*

Findings on First Examination	Follow-Up
None-to-minimal retinopathy	Annual
Mild-to-moderate NPDR and no macular edema	6–12 mo
Mild-to-moderate NPDR and early macular edema	4–6 mo
Moderate-to-severe NPDR	3–4 mo
During pregnancy	Each trimester
Very severe NPDR or early proliferative retinopathy	"Consider" treatment
High-risk proliferative retinopathy or clinically significant diabetic macular edema	"Recommend" treatment

*Following American Academy of Opthalmology Preferred Practice Pattern: Diabetic Retinopathy

from the permanent library that fundus stereo-photographs provide and are recommended in their evaluation (see Fig. 4-3). Again, fluorescein angiography is not indicated in the management of mild-to-moderate nonproliferative retinopathy, nor as a baseline measurement, if the visual acuity is consistent with the clinical examination.

MANAGEMENT OF SEVERE NONPROLIFERATIVE DIABETIC RETINOPATHY

The ETDRS has recommended that eyes of patients who have severe nonproliferative retinopathy be considered for early panretinal photocoagulation,[24] although perhaps not as urgently as eyes that have met the Diabetic Retinopathy Study (DRS) definition of high-risk retinopathy[25–27] (Fig. 4-4).

Since the DRS could not conclusively recommend either prompt treatment or waiting until retinopathy had progressed to the high-risk stages for eyes with less than high-risk diabetic retinopathy, one arm of the ETDRS was designed to look at the effect of early photocoagulation for eyes with moderate-to-severe NPDR or early proliferative disease,[2,24,28] versus deferral of treatment until high-risk retinopathy developed. They also compared the efficacy of either full-scatter panretinal photocoagulation of approximately 1200 to 1600 burns of 500-μm spot size, applied in two or more sessions, or mild-scatter panretinal photocoagulation using 400 to 650 burns, applied in a single session with otherwise similar parameters.[2,24,28] Argon blue-green or green was generally used, but krypton red was allowed if cataract or vitreous hemorrhage were present.[28] A spot size of 500 μm was set when using the Goldmann lens and usually reduced to approximately 300 μm when using the Rodenstock lens[2,28] because of the effective enlargement of the spot size on the retina.[29,30] Both strategies employed local treatment to the retina underlying surface NVE of less than two disc areas.[2,28]

Moderate and severe NPDR were defined in the ETDRS at the start of the study as previously discussed; early proliferative retinopathy is simply proliferative disease that is less than high-risk, having fewer than three retinopathy risk factors,[24,25] as defined by the DRS.[24,25] One subset of patients, who were randomized to either early panretinal photocoagulation or deferral of treatment, did not have clinically significant macular edema at baseline.[2,24] Focal photocoagulation was initiated only during follow-up if clinically significant macular edema developed. Other randomization strategies assigned eyes with less severe retinopathy (defined as mild-to-moderate NPDR) and baseline macular edema, and eyes with more severe retinopathy (defined as severe NPDR or early, less than high-risk proliferative retinopathy) and baseline macular edema to combinations of macular and scatter panretinal treatment versus deferral of photocoagulation.[2,24] These particular strategies will be discussed in Chapter 10, Special Cases.

For eyes with moderate-to-severe NPDR or early proliferative retinopathy, but no macular edema at entry, early photocoagulation resulted in lower rates of severe visual loss at each follow-up year, up until the 7-year visit (the last visit reported).[24] However, neither full nor mild early scatter treatment was significantly better than deferral of treatment in preventing moderate or severe visual loss, as the rates were low for all groups, at less than 5%. And the eyes assigned to have early full-scatter treatment were more likely to have a higher incidence of early transient moderate visual loss in the first 2 years of follow-up. This was probably partly due to the effect of panretinal photocoagulation on the development of macular edema, rather than on the eyes assigned to deferral.

But, the rate of progression to high-risk retinopathy was 19% for eyes receiving early full-scatter treatment, 27% for eyes receiving early mild-scatter treatment, and 39% for all eyes deferred at 5 years.[24] If subdivided further among moderate NPDR, severe NPDR, and early proliferative disease, certain eyes had much higher rates of progression. Eyes that had two characteristics of the 4-2-1 rule or, in

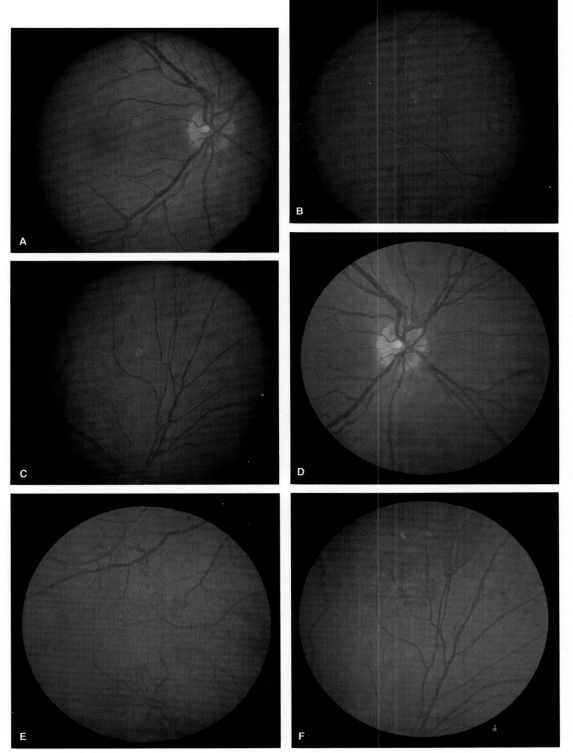

Figure 4–4 This 25-year-old white man with a 20-year history of type I diabetes showed very severe nonproliferative changes (**A–C**) according to the 4-2-1 rule, with IRMA, venous beading, and intraretinal hemorrhages throughout his fundus. The patient was followed, and the corresponding views 18 months later showed the following: (**D**) definite neovascularization of the disc greater than standard photo 10A and (**E,F**) areas of NVE had developed.

other words, very severe NPDR, developed high-risk disease at the highest rate—45% at 1 year, 65% at 3 years, and 71% at 5 years of follow-up.[5,24] This is even higher than the rate given to eyes with baseline early proliferative disease.

Guidelines for Follow-Up

Given the low rate of development of severe visual loss (less than 5%) in these eyes, the management approach must be individualized, whether treatment is given early or deferred until high-risk retinopathy develops. Still, the rate of progression to high-risk retinopathy can be quite high, especially for eyes with very severe nonproliferative retinopathy. In the DRS, over 20% of eyes assigned to immediate panretinal photocoagulation for high-risk retinopathy suffered severe visual loss, despite prompt photocoagulation.[25,27] By waiting before treating eyes with very severe nonproliferative and early proliferative retinopathy, more eyes will develop high-risk characteristics. However, the cumulative rate of severe visual loss was low in all groups in this part of the ETDRS.[24] The highest rate of severe visual loss occurred in eyes with macular edema and more severe retinopathy; in this group, this risk was reduced from 6.5% in deferral eyes to approximately 4% for all strategies of treatment.[24]

A reasonable approach then is to consider that the side effects and adverse effects of scatter treatment most probably outweigh the small benefits of early photocoagulation for eyes with moderate NPDR with a reasonably low rate of progression over 1 year.[4,5] For eyes with severe and very severe NPDR and for those with early proliferative retinopathy, the benefits of early photocoagulation should be considered (Figs. 4-5 and 4-6). Given adequate and reliable follow-up, one can wait until high-risk characteristics are approached or met before initiating treatment. Eyes with one characteristic of the 4-2-1 rule or severe nonproliferative retinopathy can be monitored clinically with frequent follow-up; early photocoagulation can be considered if, for instance, progression to the very severe stage is

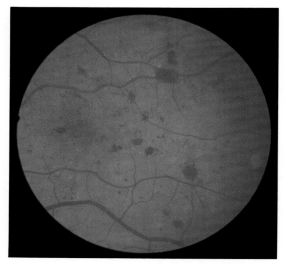

Figure 4–5 An example of severe nonproliferative diabetic retinopathy with one of the characteristics of the 4-2-1 rule: one quadrant of moderately severe IRMA.

noted with two of the 4-2-1 characteristics, as it is this stage that is associated with the highest rate of progression to high-risk retinopathy.

The fellow eye, however, can also be assessed in a comparative fashion. If the fellow eye has minimal changes and adequate follow-up is expected, one can follow this eye conservatively at first, checking for progression of disease at 3- to 4-month intervals. Once the disease appears to be worsening or high-risk

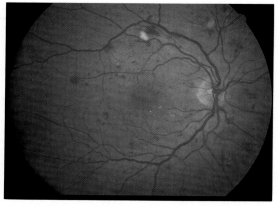

Figure 4–6 An example of very severe nonproliferative diabetic retinopathy with two of the characteristics of the 4-2-1 rule: venous beading in at least two quadrants and severe intraretinal hemorrhages and microaneurysms in four quadrants. This patient has an almost 50% chance of developing high-risk retinopathy in 1 year.

retinopathy is approached, scatter panretinal photocoagulation can be given. If the fellow eye has equivalent disease (for instance, very severe NPDR), one eye can be considered for early scatter treatment with careful clinical follow-up of the fellow nontreated eye. If it is chosen to follow the patient clinically, the patient should be evaluated at frequent intervals. If the fellow eye is significantly worse, despite previous treatment, one can assume that the eye being considered may be the only eye to provide useful vision and early and complete treatment may be indicated. Of course, if high-risk retinopathy is detected, panretinal photocoagulation should be performed expediently.

These recommendations are based on an assumption of adequate and timely follow-up. If there is any doubt about a patient's compliance with return visits, early photocoagulation for proliferative disease less than high-risk or very severe NPDR is certainly warranted. Other special circumstances for which we feel early treatment may be efficacious include pregnancy, the development of renal failure, the monocular patient, and before cataract surgery or YAG laser capsulotomy. Each of these situations has been associated with an accelerated progression of retinopathy.

We do not routinely recommend fluorescein angiography in the management of either severe nonproliferative or proliferative diabetic retinopathy. In another report by the ETDRS of angiographic factors predictive for the progression of retinopathy, greater capillary loss, capillary dilation, and fluorescein leakage correlated with a higher rate of progression from nonproliferative to proliferative disease in those eyes assigned to deferral strategies.[31] However, the ETDRS states, and we concur, that both clinical examination and correlation with color fundus photographs in the standard seven fields is sufficient for careful assessment of the stages of retinopathy. Careful clinical follow-up plays the most important role in the management of diabetic retinopathy, and the early recognition of severe NPDR and proliferative disease will permit appropriate and timely treatment, intervening in the progression of retinopathy. The parameters of panretinal photocoagulation are discussed in Chapter 6 on the management of proliferative retinopathy.

References

1. American Academy of Ophthalmology. Preferred practice pattern: diabetic retinopathy. San Francisco: American Academy of Ophthalmology; 1989.
2. Early Treatment Diabetic Retinopathy Study Research Group. ETDRS report no 7. Early treatment diabetic retinopathy study design and baseline patient characteristics. Ophthalmology 1991; 98:741–756.
3. Early Treatment Diabetic Retinopathy Study Research Group. ETDRS Report No. 10. Grading diabetic retinopathy from stereoscopic color fundus photographs—an extension of the modified Airlie House classification. Ophthalmology 1991; 98:786–806.
4. Early Treatment Diabetic Retinopathy Research Group. ETDRS Report No. 12. Fundus photographic risk factors for progression of diabetic retinopathy. Ophthalmology 1991; 98:823–833.
5. Diabetes 2000 symposium at the annual meeting of the American Academy of Ophthalmology, Anaheim, California, October, 1991.
6. Moss SE, Klein R, Kessler SD, Richie KA. Comparison between ophthalmoscopy and fundus photography of diabetic retinopathy. Ophthalmology 1985; 92:62–67.
7. Sussman EJ, Tsiaras WG, Soper KA. Diagnosis of diabetic eye disease. JAMA 1982; 247:3231–3234.
8. Palmberg P, Smith M, Waltman S, et al. The natural history of retinopathy in insulin-dependent juvenile-onset diabetes. Ophthalmology 1981; 88:613–618.
9. Javitt JC, Canner JK, Sommer A. Cost effectiveness of current approaches to the control of retinopathy in type I diabetes. Ophthalmology 1989; 96:255–264.
10. Javitt JC, Canner JK, Frank RG, et al. Detecting and treating retinopathy in patients with type I diabetes mellitus. Ophthalmology 1990; 97:483–495.
11. Javitt JC, Aiello LP, Bassi LJ, et al. Detecting and treating retinopathy in patients with type I diabetes mellitus. Ophthalmology 1991; 98:1565–1574.
12. Klein BEK, Davis MD, Segal P, et al. Diabetic retinopathy. Assessment of severity and progression. Ophthalmology 1984; 91:10–17.
13. Aiello LM, Rand LI, Briones JC, Wafai MZ, Sebestyen JG. Diabetic retinopathy in Joslin Clinic patients with adult-onset diabetes. Ophthalmology 1981; 88:619–623.
14. Klein R, Klein BEK, Syrjala SE, Davis MD, Meuer MM, Magli Y. Wisconsin Epidemiologic Study of Diabetic Retinopathy. I. Relationship of diabetic retinopathy to management of diabetes. Preliminary report. In: Diabetic renal–retinal syndrome (Vol 2). Friedman EA, L'Esperance FA, eds. New York: Grune & Stratton: 1982; 2:21–40.

15. Klein R, Klein BEK, Moss SE, Davis MD, DeMets DL. The Wisconsin Epidemiologic Study of Diabetic Retinopathy. II. Prevalence and risk of diabetic retinopathy when age at diagnosis is less than 30 years. Arch Ophthalmol 1984; 102:520–526.

16. Klein R, Klein BEK, Moss SE, Davis MD, DeMets DL. The Wisconsin Epidemiologic Study of Diabetic Retinopathy. III. Prevalence and risk of diabetic retinopathy when age at diagnosis is 30 or more years. Arch Ophthalmol 1984; 102:527–532.

17. Klein R, Klein BEK, Moss SE, Davis MD, DeMets DL. The Wisconsin Epidemiologic Study of Diabetic Retinopathy. VII. Diabetic nonproliferative retinal lesions. Ophthalmology 1987; 94:1389–1400.

18. Klein R, Klein BEK, Moss SE, Davis MD, DeMets DL. The Wisconsin Epidemiologic Study of Diabetic Retinopathy. IX. Four-year incidence and progression of diabetic retinopathy when age at diagnosis is less than 30 years. Arch Ophthalmol 1989; 107:237–243.

19. Klein R, Klein BEK, Moss SE, Davis MD, DeMets DL. The Wisconsin Epidemiologic Study of Diabetic Retinopathy. X. Four-year incidence and progression of diabetic retinopathy when age at diagnosis is 30 years or more. Arch Ophthalmol 1989; 107:244–249.

20. Klein R. The epidemiology of diabetic retinopathy: findings from the Wisconsin Epidemiologic Study of Diabetic Retinopathy. Int Ophthalmol Clin 1987; 27:230–238.

21. Klein R, Klein BEK, Neider NW, et al. Diabetic retinopathy as detected using ophthalmoscopy, a nonmydriate camera and standard fundus camera. Ophthalmology 1985; 92:485.

22. The Diabetes Retinopathy Study Research Group. DRS Report No. 6. Design, methods, and baseline results. Invest Ophthalmol Vis Sci 1981; 21:149–209.

23. Klein BEK, Moss SE, Klein R, et al. The Wisconsin Epidemiologic Study of Diabetic Retinopathy. XIII. Relationship of serum cholesterol to retinopathy and hard exudate. Ophthalmology 1991; 98:1261–1265.

24. Early Treatment Diabetes Retinopathy Study Research Group. ETDRS Report No. 9. Early photocoagulation for diabetic retinopathy. Ophthalmology 1991; 98:766–785.

25. The Diabetes Retinopathy Study Research Group. Photocoagulation treatment of proliferative diabetic retinopathy: the second report of diabetic retinopathy/vitrectomy study findings. Am J Ophthalmol 1978; 85:82–106.

26. The Diabetes Retinopathy Study Research Group. DRS Report No. 3. Four risk factors for severe visual loss in diabetic retinopathy. Arch Ophthalmol 1979; 97:654–655.

27. The Diabetes Retinopathy Study Research Group. Report No. 14. Indications for photocoagulation treatment of diabetic retinopathy. Int Ophthalmol Clin 1987; 27:239–252.

28. Early Treatment Retinopathy Study Research Group. ETDRS Report No. 3. Techniques for scatter and local photocoagulation treatment of diabetic retinopathy. Int Ophthalmol Clin 1987; 27:254–264.

29. Barr CC. Estimation of the maximum number of argon laser burns possible in panretinal photocoagulation. Am J Ophthalmol 1984; 97:697–703.

30. Reddy VM, Zamora R, Olk RJ. A comparison of the size of the burn produced by Rodenstock and Goldmann contact lenses. Am J Ophthalmol 1991; 112:212–214.

31. Early Treatment Retinopathy Study Research Group. ETDRS Report No. 13. Fluorescein angiographic risk factors for progression of diabetic retinopathy. Ophthalmology 1991; 98:834–840.

Diabetic Retinopathy: Practical Management, by R. Joseph Olk and Carol M. Lee. J.B. Lippincott Company, Philadelphia © 1993.

CHAPTER · 5

Management of Diabetic Macular Edema

EPIDEMIOLOGY

Macular edema is the leading cause of moderate visual loss in diabetic patients.[1–5] The prevalence and incidence of macular edema increases with both longer duration and overall level of concurrent retinopathy.[6–7] The Wisconsin Epidemiologic Study of Diabetic Retinopathy (WESDR) reported the prevalence of macular edema increased from 0% in insulin-taking younger-onset patients with diabetes of less than 5 years, to 29% in patients with diabetes of 20 years or longer.[6] The prevalence of macular edema ranged from 3% in older-onset patients whose diabetes was diagnosed at age 30 years or older with less than 5 years duration, to 28% in patients with diabetes of 20 years or longer. In general, macular edema was seen more frequently in insulin-dependent older-onset patients in the first few years after diagnosis of diabetes (Fig. 5-1). In addition, when correlating the relative level of retinopathy with the presence of macular edema 2% to 6% of patients with background retinopathy had coexistent macular edema—the longer the duration, the higher the rate (Fig. 5-2). Of patients with proliferative retinopathy, 20% to 63% had

macular edema; the higher percentages in each category were noted with longer duration of diabetes and worse concurrent diabetic retinopathy.[6]

From studies of the 4-year incidence of diabetic retinopathy, the incidence of any macular edema and clinically significant macular edema was highest in the older-onset insulin-dependent and younger-onset subsets of patients with overall 4-year incidence of 8% and 5%, respectively, for the older-onset insulin-dependent patients, and 8% and 4%, respectively, for the younger-onset group of patients.[7] These figures were lower in the older-onset non–insulin-dependent subset, with corresponding incidence of 3% and 1%, lowering the total incidence in the overall group of older-onset patients (Fig. 5-3). The 4-year incidence of macular edema was directly related to the severity of diabetic retinopathy at the baseline examination. At 4 years, approximately 1% of both younger-onset and older-onset patients without baseline retinopathy had macular edema; about 10% of younger-onset and 6% of older-onset patients with baseline minimal background retinopathy had macular edema; about 15% of younger-onset and 20% of older-onset patients with baseline moderate back-

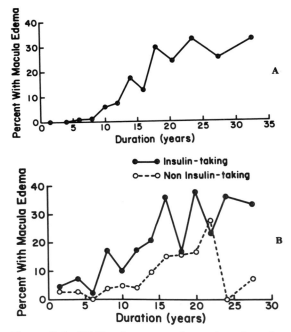

ground retinopathy disease had macular edema; and about 23% of younger-onset and 24% of older-onset patients with preproliferative retinopathy had macular edema.

The WESDR is a population-based study and may underestimate the number of patients with macular edema when compared with the number of patients in a diabetes clinic. Clinic-based studies more frequently report a higher prevalence and incidence of macular edema in older-onset patients,[8,9] whereas the WESDR reports an overall higher prevalence and incidence in the younger-onset groups. This discrepancy is reflected by the fact that there are many more older-onset diabetic patients than younger-onset[10] and that visual impairment caused by macular edema is more frequently experienced in older-onset patients who are, therefore, more likely to be examined in a diabetes clinic.[11,12] When the data from the WESDR was reviewed and projections were made concerning the risk of developing new macular edema, they found that most new cases of either any macular edema or of clinically significant macular edema would be found in the older-onset patient population.

Figure 5–1 (**A**) The frequency of macular edema by duration of diabetes in years for insulin-taking younger-onset persons. (**B**) The frequency of macular edema by duration of diabetes for insulin- and non-insulin–taking older-onset persons. [From Klein R, et al. The Wisconsin Epidemiologic Study of Diabetic Retinopathy: IV. Diabetic macular edema. (Published courtesy of Ophthalmology 1984; 91:1464–1475.)]

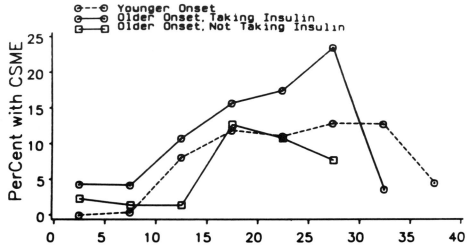

Figure 5–2 Frequency of clinically significant macular edema (CSDME, as defined in the ETDRS) by duration of diabetes (in years) in younger-onset persons taking insulin (*n* = 996) and older-onset persons taking insulin (*n* = 674) or not taking insulin (*n* = 696), who participated in the Wisconsin Epidemiologic Study of Diabetic Retinopathy, 1980–1982. (From Klein R, et al. The epidemiology of diabetic retinopathy: findings from the Wisconsin Epidemiologic Study of Diabetic Retinopathy. Int Ophthalmol Clin 1987; 27:230–238 with permission.)

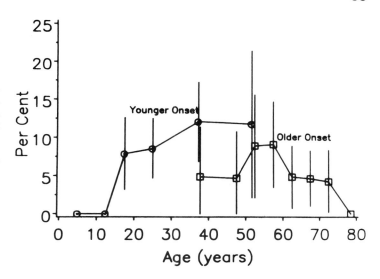

Figure 5–3 The incidence of macular edema by age at the baseline examination for younger- and older-onset persons. The solid vertical bars represent 95% confidence intervals around the rates. [From Klein R, et al. The Wisconsin Study of Diabetic Retinopathy. XI. The incidence of macular edema. (Published courtesy of Ophthalmology 1989; 96: 1501–1510.)]

EARLY TREATMENT DIABETIC RETINOPATHY STUDY

Numerous clinical trials have reported the efficacy of laser photocoagulation in the treatment of diabetic macular edema,[1,13–19] employing focal, modified grid, or grid photocoagulation. The Early Treatment Diabetic Retinopathy Study (ETDRS) has stated that prompt photocoagulation of clinically significant diabetic macular edema reduces visual loss by one-half,[13,15] the diagnosis being based on the clinical examination, regardless of visual acuity, and not on angiographic findings (Fig. 5-4).

Slit-lamp biomicroscopy is used to assess the overall thickness of the macula and the overall area affected. Retinal thickening is probably most easily appreciated with contact lens biomicroscopy, using either the posterior pole contact lens or the Goldmann three-mirror lens. The hand-held 60-, 78-, and 90-diopter lenses are quite useful, especially when there is significant thickening; however, in early or borderline cases the contact lens examination is probably more sensitive.[20]

Thickening of the normal retina is generally judged to appear approximately twice the diameter of a major retinal vein at the optic disc margin; this is usually considered to be the *reference thickness.*[21] At the center of the fovea, the retina is normally flat, appearing to be directly apposed to the retinal pigment epithe-

lium. In the most recent definitions published by the ETDRS, grading for diabetic retinopathy characteristics in field 2, as defined in the seven standard fields of the Modified Airlie House classification, has been expanded.[21] Thickening can be subdivided into three locations relative to the center of the macula. These locations include the following:

1. All of field 2 (centered on the macula)

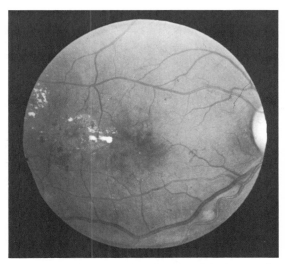

Figure 5–4 An example of early diabetic macular edema that is not clinically significant. Thickening and exudate are located farther than 500 μm from the center of the macula. We did not obtain an angiogram, as the patient did not require treatment. She was asked to return in 4 months for repeat evaluation.

2. The area of retina within one disc diameter of the center of the macula
3. The center of the macula

However, the definition of clinical significance is unchanged by this additional qualification.

The treatment itself is dependent on the type of leakage that is felt to cause the retinal thickening. The ETDRS employed a treatment strategy that addressed, primarily, focal leakage and, secondarily, diffuse leakage. Their protocol required that all focal points of leakage located between 500 μm and two disc diameters (=3000 μm) be treated directly. At first, 50- to 100-μm spots at 0.1-second duration with argon blue-green or green alone were used to effect a whitening of the microaneurysm. Repeat

focal burns were sometimes needed,[13,15] especially in microaneurysms larger than 40 μm.

In the ETDRS, focal lesions located 300 to 500 μm from the center of the macula could be treated if the visual acuity was 20/40 or worse and if the treating ophthalmologist did not believe that laser photocoagulation of these lesions would destroy the remaining perifoveal capillary network. Focal treatment between 300 and 500 μm from the center of the macula was optional at the initial session, but required at the follow-up sessions if the aforementioned criteria were met. Most focal leaks are caused by individual microaneurysms, although short, diseased capillary segments may show local leakage. Red spots not angiographically evident, but believed to be microaneurysms by

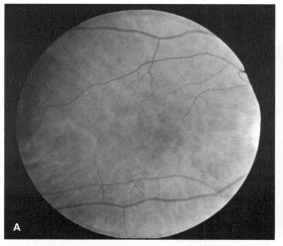

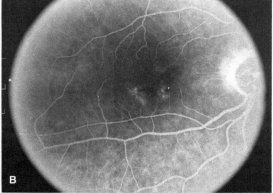

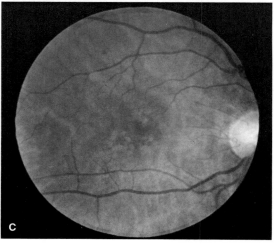

Figure 5–5   A 74-year-old white man with adult-onset diabetes of 10-years duration presented with (**A**) clinically significant diabetic macular edema and visual acuity of 20/20. (**B**) Fluorescein angiography revealed focal areas of leakage that (**C**) were treated with focal laser photocoagulation.

their configuration and not intraretinal hemorrhages, could be treated focally. Clusters of microaneurysms could be treated with larger spot sizes of 200 to 500 μm, but confluent treatment such as this was not recommended within 750 μm of the center of the macula (Fig. 5-5).

In the ETDRS, grid treatment consisted of burns of 50- to 200-μm spot size of lighter intensity than that required for panretinal photocoagulation, placed one burn width apart, at 0.1-second duration. This treatment was applied to areas of diffuse leakage or capillary nonperfusion. The grid treatment could be placed in the papillomacular bundle, but outside 500 μm from the edge of the optic disc and not within 500 μm of the center of the macula (Fig. 5-6).

Follow-up treatment was recommended in their protocol if residual clinically significant macular edema with treatable lesions was seen during clinical examination, at 4 months after initial treatment, and at 4-month intervals between treatments. Fluorescein angiography

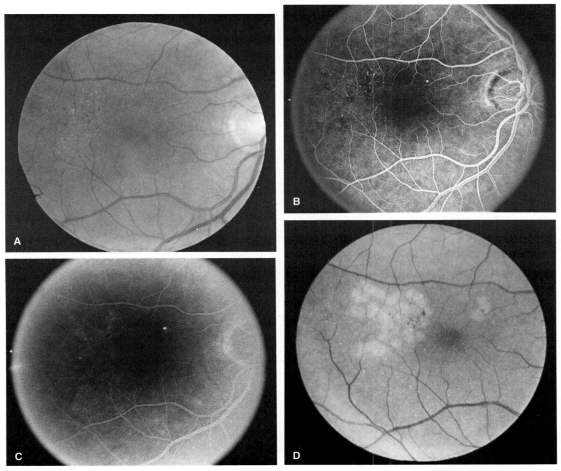

Figure 5–6 A 59-year-old white woman with type II non-insulin–dependent diabetes presented with (**A**) nonproliferative diabetic retinopathy and clinically significant diabetic macular edema. There was an area of macular thickening of one disc area within 500 μm of the center of the macula, and drusen scattered throughout the posterior pole. (**B,C**) Fluorescein angiography showed numerous microaneurysms that leaked focally and areas of diffuse leakage superotemporal to the fovea. (**D**) A combination of focal and grid treatment was applied to the areas of microaneurysms and retinal thickening temporal to the FAZ and, in addition, focal treatment was applied to microaneurysms superonasal to the FAZ.

was generally repeated for guidance in treatment. All focal leaks outside 500 μm from the center of the macula were treated. Focal leaks within 500 μm of the center of the macula were treated if it was felt that such treatment would not destroy the remaining perifoveal capillary network and the visual acuity was 20/40 or less. Grid treatment was, in general, not reapplied to areas previously treated with grid.

MODIFIED-GRID PHOTOCOAGULATION

The use and efficacy of grid treatment has been studied in numerous trials.[22–25] Modified grid photocoagulation, as described by Olk[18,19,26,27] employs primarily grid treatment to areas of diffuse leakage, with occasional focal treatment of focal leakage located either within or outside the areas of diffuse edema. *Diffuse diabetic macular edema* is defined as retinal thickening of two or more disc areas *and* involving some portion of the foveal avascular zone (FAZ), with or without cystoid macular edema. The definition is similar to that of the ETDRS for more advanced cases of clinically significant diabetic macular edema, but must involve the FAZ.

Visual results at 2- and 3-year follow-up with modified grid treatment are comparable with the ETDRS; modified grid treatment appears effective in preventing moderate visual loss in patients with diffuse diabetic macular edema.[18,19,26,27] After following patients for up to 5 years, Lee and Olk found that 85% of patients treated with modified grid remained the same or had improvement of vision at each annual follow-up visit.[27] The majority of eyes maintained their initial visual acuity within two lines of change throughout follow-up with 61%, 62%, and 56% remaining the same at 3-, 4-, and 5-year follow-up visits, respectively. Also, the presence of cystoid macular edema, which frequently accompanies diffuse diabetic macular edema, did not adversely affect the visual outcome of the treated eyes.[18,19,27] Resolution of the central zone of edema involving the FAZ was noted in 84% of patients during 5-year follow-up.[27]

Practical Guidelines

When eyes are determined by clinical examination to have central retinal thickening, consistent with clinically significant diabetic macular edema, and the decision to treat has been made, a fluorescein angiogram should be obtained. If the angiogram reveals mainly diffuse leakage with only occasional focal leaking microaneurysms, modified grid treatment is applied. If the angiogram reveals mainly focal

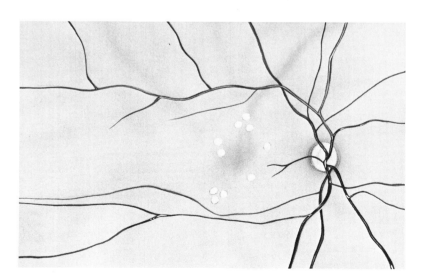

Figure 5–7 Artist's illustration of typical focal treatment to individual leaking microaneurysms. The laser burns are of 100-μm spot size.

Figure 5–8 Artist's illustration of typical modified grid laser photocoagulation treatment. Two to three rows of 100-μm spots are applied 100-μm apart in the parafoveal region up to and including the edge of the foveal avascular zone. Then 150- or 200-μm spots are applied 200-μm apart throughout all areas of retinal thickening or areas of nonperfusion. [From Olk RJ. Argon green (514 nm) versus krypton red (647 nm) modified grid laser photocoagulation for diffuse diabetic macular edema. (Published courtesy of Ophthalmology 1990; 97:1101–1113.)]

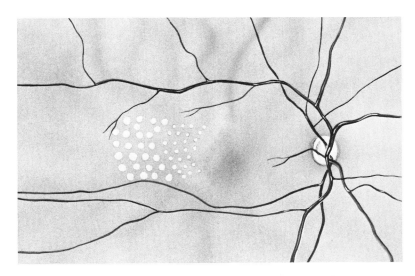

leakage, focal treatment is applied directly to the leaking microaneurysms (Fig. 5-7). The fluorescein angiogram should be projected on a viewer, such as a Topcon, or on a screen in easy view of the laser surgeon. Modified grid is applied using two or three rows of 100-μm spots to all areas of perifoveal thickening up to and including the edge of the FAZ; these initial spots are placed 100-μm apart. Then, 150- to 200-μm spots are placed approximately 200 μm apart to the remaining areas of retinal thickening and capillary nonperfusion (Fig. 5-8). Focal leaks outside or within the zones of diffuse leakage are treated with 100- to 150-μm

spots to achieve a mild whitening of the microaneurysm (Figs. 5-9 through 5-11).

The endpoint of each laser burn used in a grid pattern is a light-intensity burn just barely visible at the level of the outer retina or retinal pigment epithelium. The endpoint of each focal laser burn is slightly darker in intensity with moderate whitening of the microaneurysm. However, the authors no longer advocate the goal of closing the microaneurysm, as described in the ETDRS protocol. Nor do we repeatedly treat the microaneurysm for complete obliteration or pretreat the microaneurysm with first a 100-μm spot followed by a 50-μm spot; 100- to

Figure 5–9 Artist's illustration of modified grid treatment that includes grid pattern to areas of retinal thickening or areas of nonperfusion, as well as focal treatment with additional 100- to 150-μm spots applied in areas of obvious focal leakage. [From Olk RJ. Argon green (514 nm) versus krypton red (647 nm) modified grid laser photocoagulation for diffuse diabetic macular edema. (Published courtesy of Ophthalmology 1990; 97:1101–1113.)]

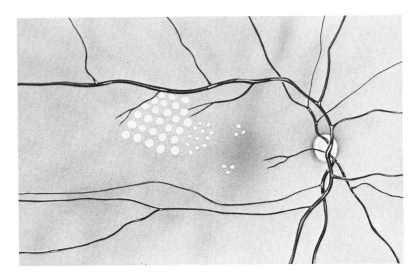

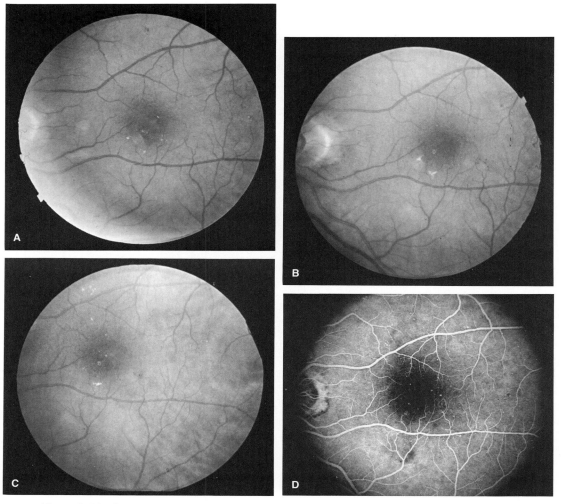

Figure 5–10   A 57-year-old white man with insulin-dependent type I diabetes of 15-years duration presented with (**A**) early nonproliferative retinopathy consisting of hard exudates and microaneurysms, but retinal thickening farther than 500 μm from the center of the fovea. (**B**) He was followed at 4-month intervals during which time visual acuity remained the same and exudates increased slightly. (**C**) One year after initial presentation, the central macula is now thickened with cystic change. (**D,E**) Macular photocoagulation was advised and fluorescein angiography was obtained for use as a guide during treatment. Fluorescein angiograms showed the diffuse leakage with central cystoid. (**F**) Modified grid was applied to all areas of retinal thickening. (**G**) Nine months after treatment, the macula is completely flat, with no residual edema.

(continued)

150-μm focal laser spots are applied at 0.1-second duration with the argon or krypton wavelengths.

In focal photocoagulation, the lighter-intensity burns provide adequate stimulation for endothelial cell replication, which theoretically works to close the microaneurysm.[28] It is not

known specifically how laser photocoagulation works to reduce or eliminate diabetic macular edema. The diffuse type of macular edema may be a product of both inner and outer blood–retinal barrier damage, as discussed briefly in Chapter 2. The replication of the endothelial cells of the inner blood–retinal barrier may

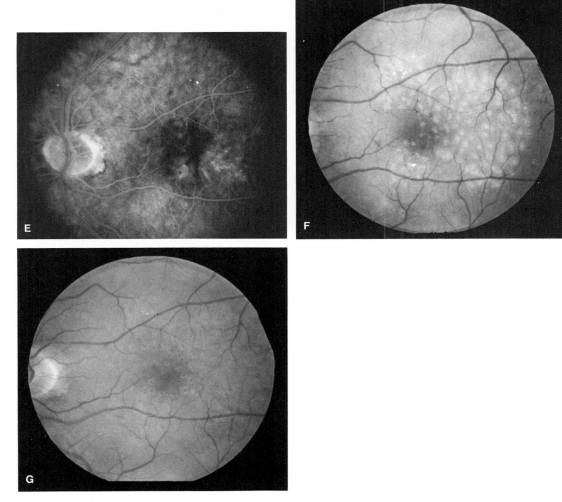

Figure 5–10 (continued)

be enhanced secondarily by laser-induced changes in the outer blood–retinal barrier, such as the retinal pigment epithelium.[28] This replication may close the microaneurysm itself or may enhance or reestablish the function of the inner blood–retinal barrier.

The retinal pigment epithelium undergoes both anatomic remodeling and functional restoration in cynomolgus monkeys treated with mild argon laser photocoagulation.[29] After Hunter dystrophic rats were treated with pulsed ruby laser, phagocytosis of subretinal debris occurring normally in these strains by retinal pigment epithelial cells was seen.[30] It is

possible that some factors are elaborated by the retinal pigment epithelium to enable repair of the endothelial cells within the inner blood–retinal barrier and for subsequent resolution or amelioration of the edema.

Another theory is that the grid laser reduces the demand for oxygen by destroying the outer retina permitting an increased supply of oxygen to the inner retinal layers.[31] The retinal pigment epithelium has been shown experimentally to account for two-thirds of the retinal demand for oxygen.[32] Once the abnormal retinal pigment epithelium cells that may be causing the diffuse edema and be consuming the

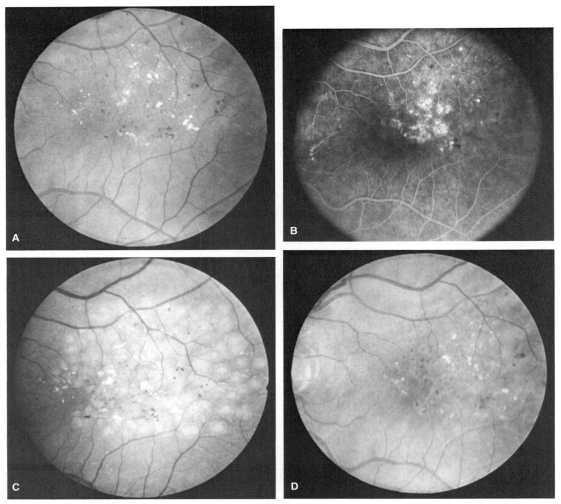

Figure 5–11　A 59-year-old white woman with non-insulin–dependent diabetes presented with (**A,B**) diffuse diabetic macular edema superotemporally in her left eye. (**C**) Modified grid was performed to the areas of retinal thickening up to and including the edge of the FAZ. (**D**) Three months later central edema had resolved, although residual exudates are still noted. (**E,F**) Fluorescein angiography revealed no residual central leakage. (**G,H**) Three years after initial presentation, visual acuity was 20/25 and there was no residual macular edema.

(continued)

most oxygen are destroyed by photocoagulation, the inner retina may receive a greater supply of oxygen, enabling more oxygen to diffuse from the choroid to the inner retina, thereby diminishing the ischemia and possibly reducing the stimulus for angiogenesis factors.[32] Or the additional metabolic support may enable the replication of a functional inner blood–retinal barrier. Our lighter treatment, in addition to being adequate for endothelial re-

pair, capillary closure, and stimulation of reparative processes by the outer retina–retinal pigment epithelium–choriocapillaris complex, may result in fewer paracentral scotomata, a known side effect of macular treatment.

Given these possible hypotheses for the mechanism of laser photocoagulation, modified grid photocoagulation differs from focal laser treatment in its extent and goal. Instead of individual microaneurysmal closure, the

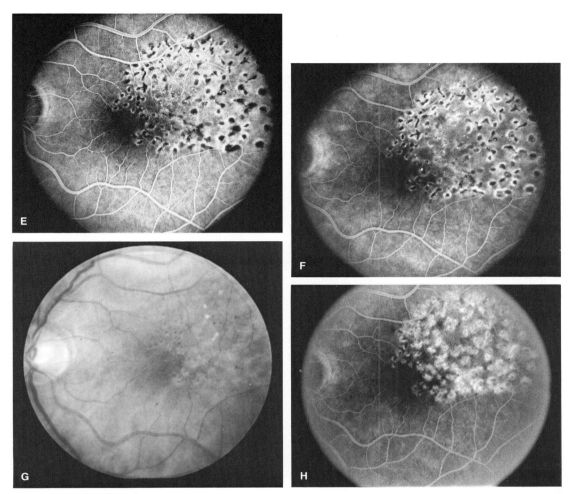

Figure 5–11 (continued)

grid pattern covers more completely areas of capillary dysfunction, presumably causing diffuse edema. At the same time, more extensive photocoagulation of the retinal pigment epithelium and outer retinal layers may enhance the reparative processes. For focal leakage, however, the direct delivery of laser to the microaneurysm should be sufficient for the initiation of the reparative processes, without actual physical closure of the microaneurysm.

In the modified grid, all grid treatments are given at 0.1-second duration, using either argon green or krypton red wavelength. The modified grid is performed usually under topical, but rarely under retrobulbar, anesthesia. In a recent randomized clinical trial, Olk showed that there were no statistically significant differences between eyes treated with an argon green versus a krypton red modified grid for diffuse diabetic macular edema relative to reduction or elimination of macular edema, improvement or worsening of visual acuity, number of treatments, or effect on visual field.[19,26,33] Additionally, argon pure green and krypton red have the added benefit of sparing the nerve fiber layer compared with the argon blue-green wavelength.[34] This is clinically manifested by fewer subjective complaints of paracentral scotomata with argon green or krypton red treatment than with argon blue-green.[19,26,33] In general, we use argon green for macular treatments; however, krypton red is useful in the presence of cataract or vitreous hemorrhage.

Modified grid photocoagulation is applied only to areas of retinal thickening or capillary nonperfusion seen on the clinical biomicroscopic examination and confirmed on fluorescein angiography. Treatment is not routinely applied to the entire posterior pole. For example, an area of diffuse retinal edema located temporal to and involving the FAZ is treated with a grid pattern in that temporal region; obvious microaneurysms that are located either within or outside the zone of diffuse thickening are treated focally. Treatment is applied up to and including the edge of the FAZ, but not within it. We do not treat any microaneurysm that is located within the FAZ.

Indication for Supplemental Treatment

Supplemental treatments are usually performed at 3 to 4 months between each session.

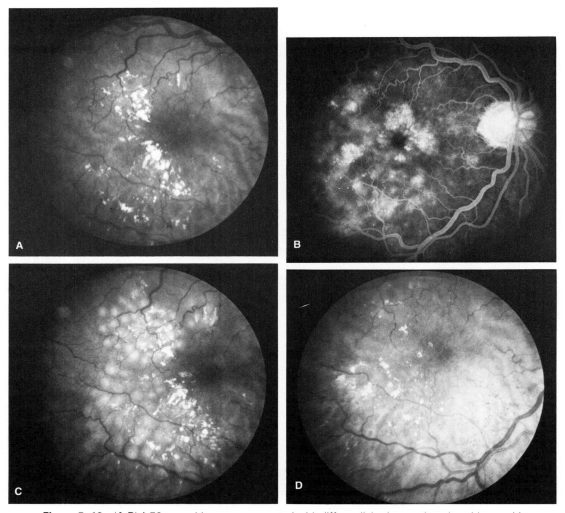

Figure 5–12   (**A,B**) A 72-year-old woman presented with diffuse diabetic maculopathy with cystoid macular edema in her right eye. Visual acuity was 20/63. (**C**) She received modified grid laser photocoagulation. (**D,E**) Three months after the first treatment, central retinal thickening and cystoid macular edema persisted, and (**F**) the eye received supplemental modified grid treatment. (**G,H**) Three months later, the central retinal thickening resolved and visual acuity was 20/50.

(continued)

Supplemental treatment is indicated if residual central thickening involving the FAZ is noted on follow-up clinical examination spaced at 3- to 4-month intervals. Once the central thickening is resolved, no further supplemental treatments are required unless or until the central FAZ becomes thickened again. On the average, patients will require two modified grid treatments before retinal thickening involving the central FAZ is eliminated.[27] However, as it is known that each additional supplemental treatment causes a cumulative decrease in the paracentral visual field, our goal is to eliminate the residual central thickening;[33] residual thickening outside the central FAZ is no longer

an indication for supplemental treatment (Figs. 5-12 through 5-14).

Practical Guidelines

The settings for supplemental modified grid are similar to those used for the original initial treatment. We generally use the same wavelength for supplemental treatments that was used in the initial treatment. Treatment is applied to areas of retinal thickening involving the FAZ, regardless of whether treatment had been applied to that area before. A new fluorescein angiogram is obtained before supplemental treatment.

(continued on page 66)

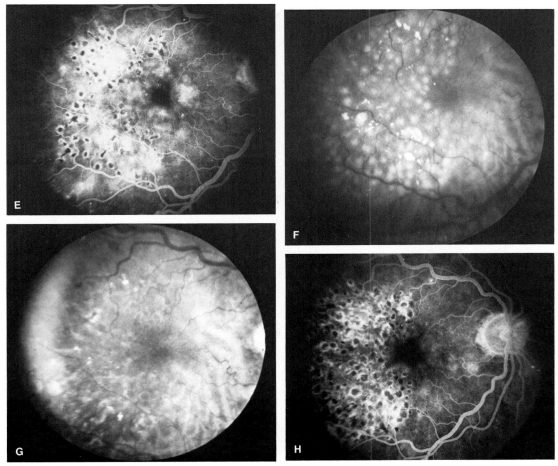

Figure 5–12 (continued)

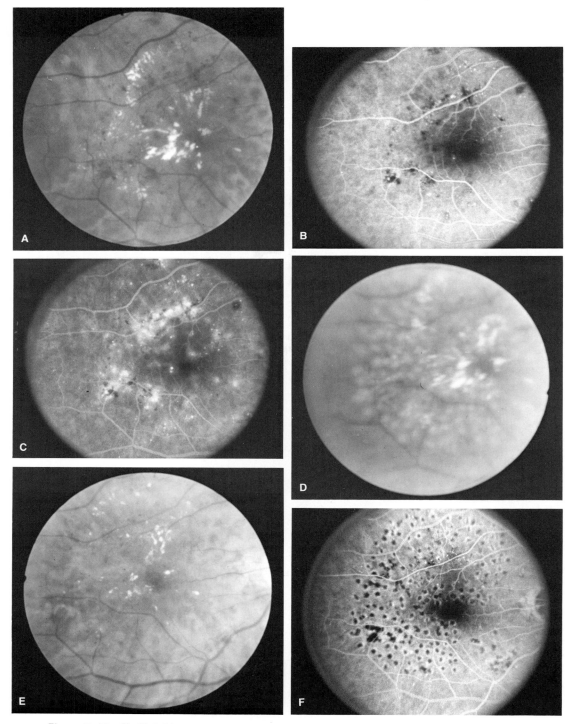

Figure 5–13 (**A–C**) A 62-year-old woman presented with diffuse diabetic macular edema in her right eye. Her visual acuity was 20/40. (**D**) The patient received modified grid laser photocoagulation. (**E–G**) Four months later there was still residual central macular edema. (**H**) The patient received supplemental modified grid photocoagulation to areas of residual retinal thickening. (**I–K**) Three months after supplemental treatment, there was some residual edema superior to the macula, but the central macula itself appeared flat. (**L**) Three years later the area of residual retinal thickening superiorly had completely resolved and visual acuity was 20/20.

64

(continued)

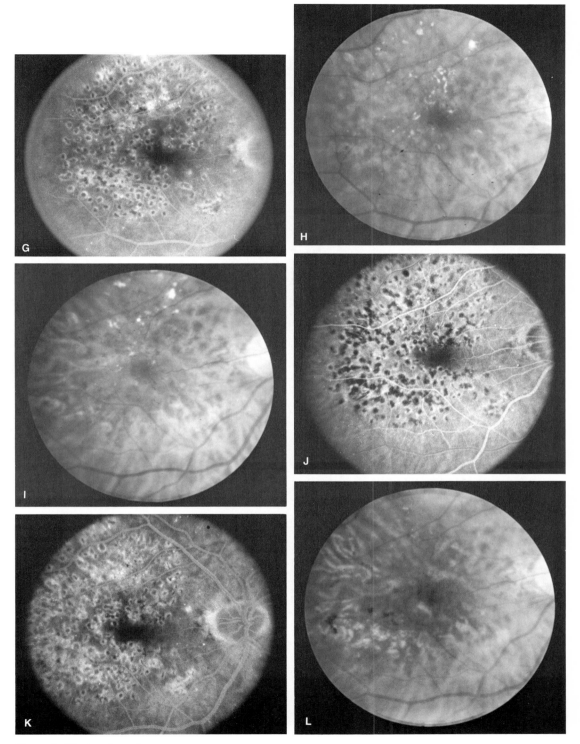

Figure 5–13 (continued)

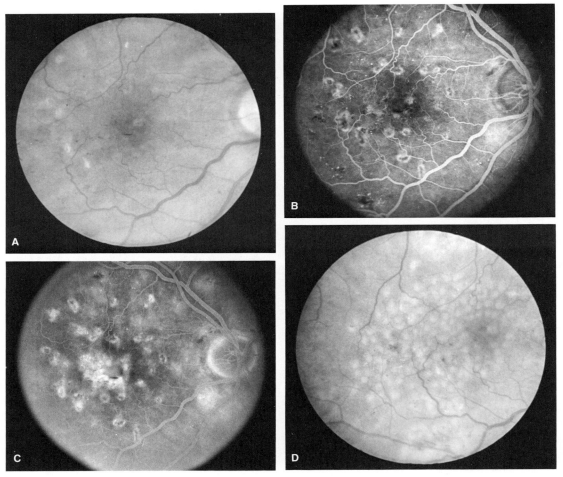

Figure 5–14 A 64-year-old white woman, with a 26-year history of type I diabetes, was referred to us having had previous focal treatment for macular edema. She complained of a recent decrease in visual acuity and was seen with (**A**) central macular thickening. (**B,C**) Fluorescein angiography revealed diffuse leakage with central cystoid. Previous focal photocoagulation scars were also noted. (**D**) Modified grid laser photocoagulation was performed to all areas of retinal thickening. (**E**) Four months later there was residual central retinal thickening. (**F,G**) Fluorescein angiography showed central macular leakage with cystoid, and (**H**) supplemental grid treatment was performed. (**I–K**) Four months later there was still residual central macular thickening, and (**L**) she received another supplemental treatment. (**M–O**) Six months later there was no evidence of retinal thickening, and visual acuity remained stable at 20/50 as it had throughout the course of this patient's treatment.

(continued)

If the eye shows predominantly focal leakage, focal photocoagulation, as described by the ETDRS with our few previously mentioned modifications, is advised. Again, a recent fluorescein angiogram should be projected either on a screen or on a viewer to guide in the treatment. The power of the focal laser burn should be directed at producing a mild-to-moderate white burn at the level of the microaneurysms; however, we do not try to obliterate the microaneurysm and do not pretreat the microaneu-

(continued on page 71)

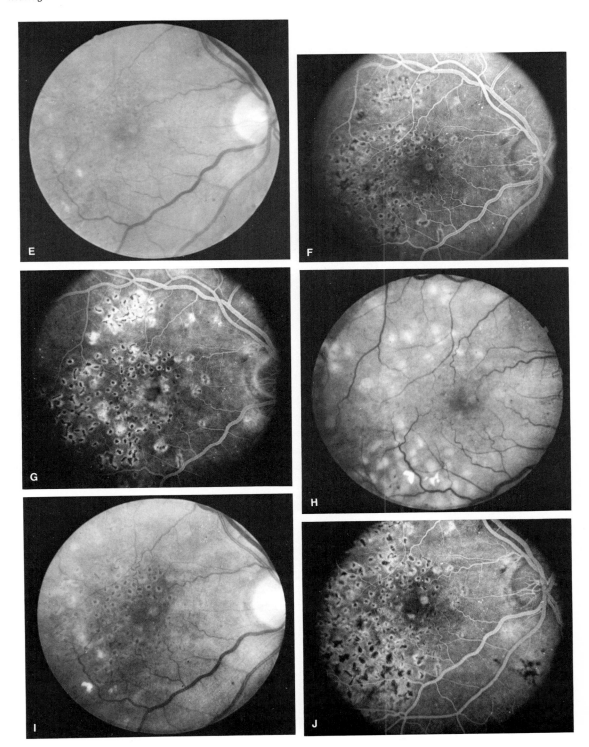

Figure 5–14 (continued)

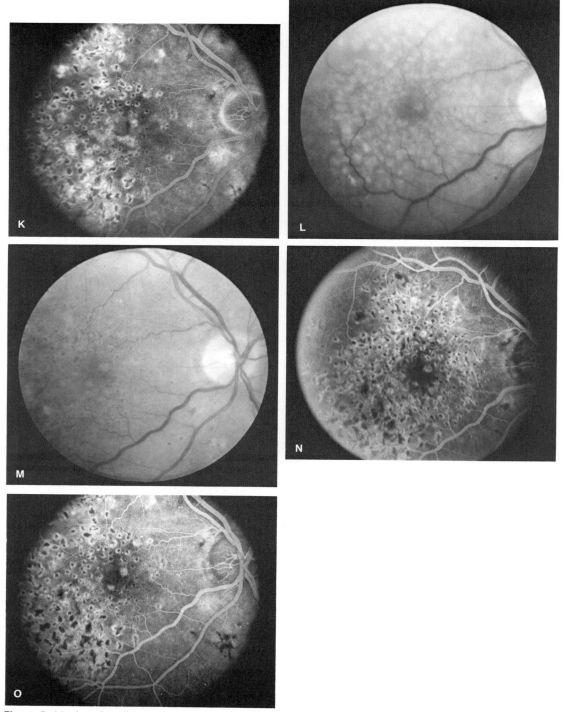

Figure 5–14 (continued)

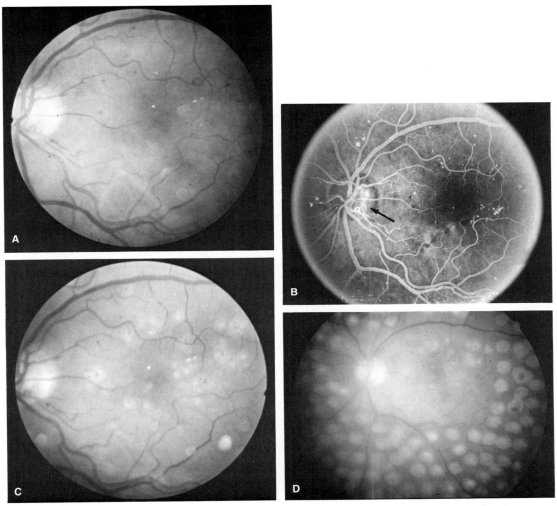

Figure 5–15 A 62-year-old white man with type II insulin-dependent diabetes of 3-years duration presented with (**A**) early clinically significant diabetic macular edema and early NVD equal to standard photo 10A. Visual acuity was 20/25. (**B**) Fluorescein angiography showed NVD (*arrow*) and focal microaneurysms. (**C**) The patient received combined focal macular treatment and (**D**) scatter panretinal photocoagulation to the left eye in one session. (**E**) The proliferative disease regressed, but there was persistent central edema. (**F,G**) Fluorescein angiography showed residual leakage from microaneurysms and central cystic change. (**H**) Supplemental focal treatment was applied to the leaking microaneurysms. (**I**) Six months later, visual acuity was 20/50, and there was no central retinal thickening. (**J,K**) Two years later, the patient had recurrent central thickening, with focal leakage from microaneurysms, and (**L**) a second supplemental focal treatment was given. (**M**) Four months after this, visual acuity was 20/50 and there was no evidence of macular edema on clinical examination, (**N**) which was confirmed by fluorescein angiography.

(continued)

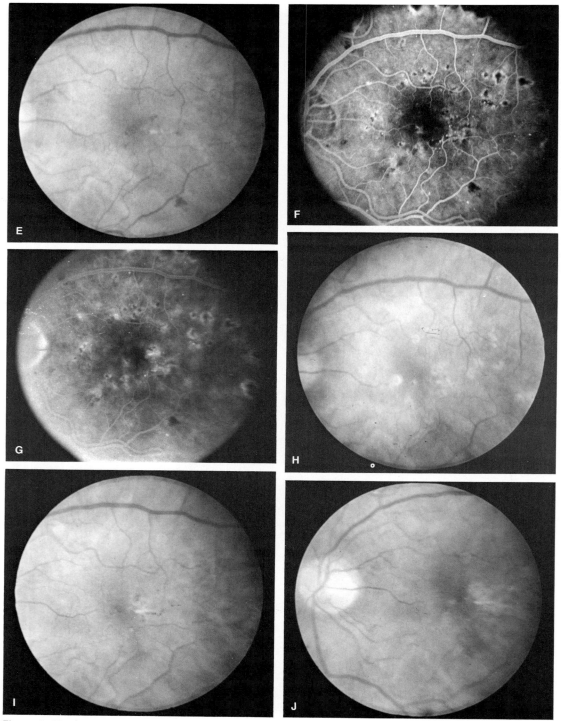

Figure 5–15   (continued)

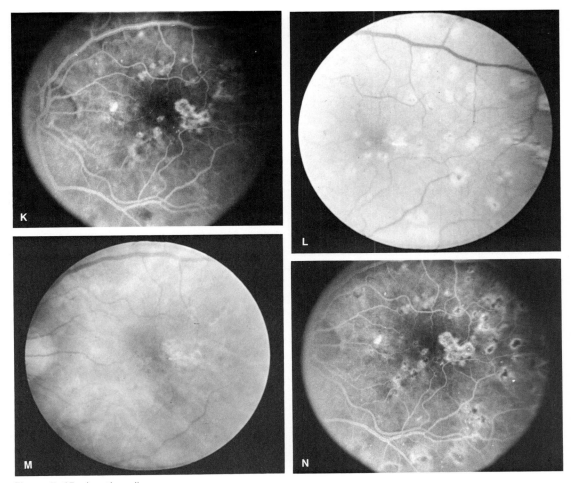

Figure 5–15 (continued)

rysm with a larger 100-μm spot followed by a 50-μm spot. The spot size is from 100 μm to 150 μm at 0.1-second duration for both argon green and krypton red focal treatments.

Red spots that appear to be microaneurysms despite their lack of filling on angiography are treated, but those that appear to be intraretinal hemorrhages are not treated. Clusters of microaneurysms should not be treated with overlapping confluent burns, but rather, with a grid-type pattern to avoid paracentral scotomata. Treatment is brought up to the edge of the FAZ but not within it and can be extended into the papillomacular bundle. Scanning of the treated areas to check for reperfusion of the microaneurysms is not done because our goal is not to close the microaneurysm, but, rather, to deliver just enough energy to stimulate the natural pathophysiologic mechanisms to effect closure.

Guidelines for Follow-Up

Follow-up is scheduled at 3- to 4-month intervals. If central thickening persists or if the patient meets the ETDRS definition of clinical significance, repeat treatments are indicated. The

(continued on page 74)

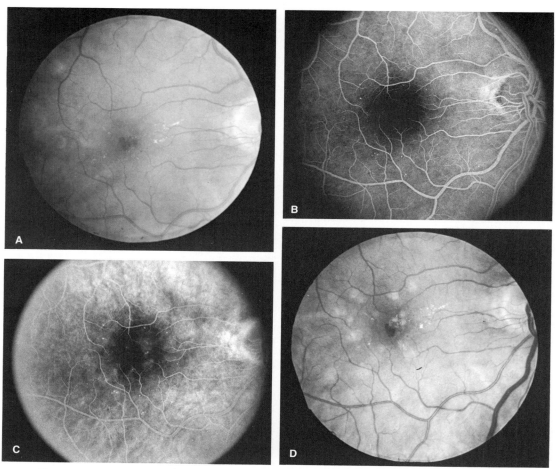

Figure 5–16   A 62-year-old man presented with (**A**) clinically significant diabetic macular edema, and visual acuity was 20/50. (**B,C**) Fluorescein angiography revealed focal areas of leakage, and (**D**) focal laser photocoagulation was performed. (**E**) Four months later, central macular edema had resolved and the patient had no residual retinal thickening, with visual acuity of 20/20. (**F,G**) Fluorescein angiography showed characteristic hypofluorescent spots surrounded by hyperfluorescence typical of laser photocoagulation scars, without retinal vascular leakage. (**H**) The patient remained stable over the next 2 years, but then presented with recurrent macular edema affecting the central macula. (**I,J**) Fluorescein angiography showed recurrent leakage, with central cystic change. (**K**) The patient received modified grid laser photocoagulation and the superonasal focal leaks were treated with focal laser photocoagulation. (**L**) Nine months later no residual macular edema was present and visual acuity remained stable at 20/50.

(continued)

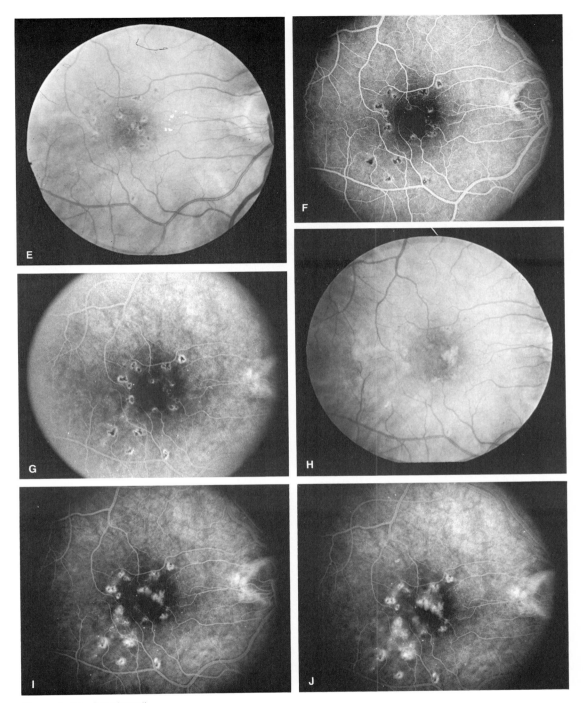

Figure 5–16 (continued)

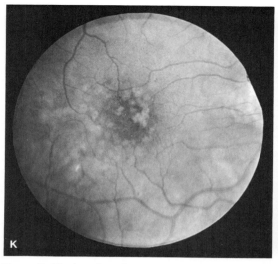

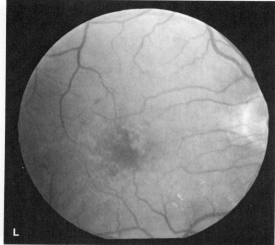

Figure 5–16   (continued)

pattern of treatment used should be based on which type is more preponderant, focal or diffuse leakage, as determined by angiography. If the patient has good vision (visual acuity of 20/25 or better) or improved vision with significant reduction in edema, mild residual thickening of the central FAZ can be followed closely without immediate retreatment. Fundus photography immediately following treatment can be useful for documentation (Figs. 5-15 and 5-16).

Patients who are seen with clinically significant macular edema or macular edema greater than two disc areas and involving the FAZ should be considered for treatment, be it focal, grid, or modified grid. However, if a patient has very good vision (e.g., 20/20 visual acuity) with early clinically significant macular edema, without central involvement, it would not be unreasonable to offer a choice of follow-up or treatment, as the rate of visual loss is reasonably low, even without treatment.[13–15] But, if it appears that the edema is progressing toward the center of the macula with serial examinations (here, fundus stereophotographs are especially valuable, as documentation allows careful comparison), or if most of the treatable lesions are outside of 500 μm from the center of the macula,[14,15] the decision may be weighed in favor of photocoagulation. The known side

effects of macular treatment, namely, paracentral scotomata,[13,33,35] and the immediate risk of vision loss owing to a misplaced laser spot, especially when treating within 500 μm of the center of the fovea, need to be kept in mind when considering the treatment of eyes with good visual acuity. Nevertheless, those eyes with central involvement or clinically significant macular edema with good visual acuity should be considered for photocoagulation.

In selected cases with extensive macular leakage, it may be difficult to ascertain exactly where the edge of the FAZ is. In these patients, it is better to treat conservatively in the initial session of macular photocoagulation, knowing that the patient will most likely require supplemental treatments. The edema and leakage should have decreased somewhat after the first treatment session, permitting a clearer view of the FAZ at the supplemental session, if needed. At this point, treatment can be brought up to the edge of the FAZ more easily, but never within this zone.

Patients who are seen with less than severe nonproliferative retinopathy and macular edema that does not meet clinical significance should be evaluated again at 4- to 6-month intervals to assess the progression of their macular edema. Neither treatment nor fluorescein

(continued on page 79)

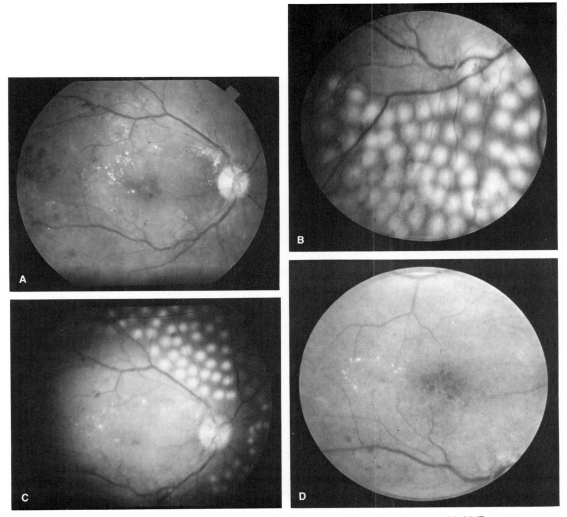

Figure 5–17 A 30-year-old woman presented with early proliferative disease, with NVE greater than one-half disc area. She had multiple areas of intraretinal lipid, but no clinically significant macular edema. (**A**) In the past, the patient had been noncompliant with follow-up, so panretinal treatment was recommended for her early proliferative retinopathy. (**B,C**) The patient received panretinal photocoagulation in two sessions, and over the next year, the patient received one additional session of panretinal photocoagulation for new preretinal hemorrhage. (**D–F**) Her proliferative disease stabilized, but she then developed diffuse diabetic macular edema, with cystoid macular edema. (**G**) Modified grid laser photocoagulation was given. (**H–J**) Three months later she had residual central macular edema with cystoid and (**K**) was treated with supplemental modified grid. Over the next year, at each of her follow-up visits, she had persistent central edema with cystoid edema for which she received three additional supplemental grid treatments. (**L–N**) The fundus photographs and fluorescein angiogram taken before her second supplemental treatment and (**O–Q**) those taken before her fourth supplemental treatment, at which time she still had diffuse diabetic macular edema and cystoid macular edema are shown. (**R**) She received a fourth supplemental modified grid treatment and (**S–U**) after five macular treatments, both the central edema and the cystoid macular edema completely resolved and visual acuity was stable at 20/80.

(continued)

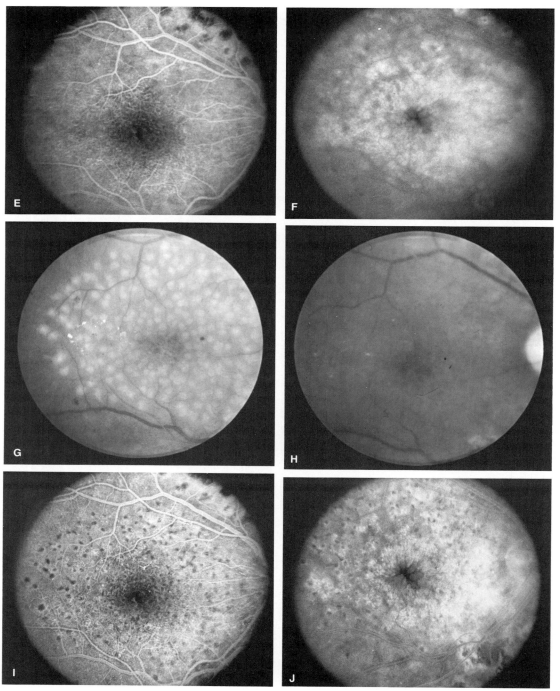

Figure 5–17   (continued)

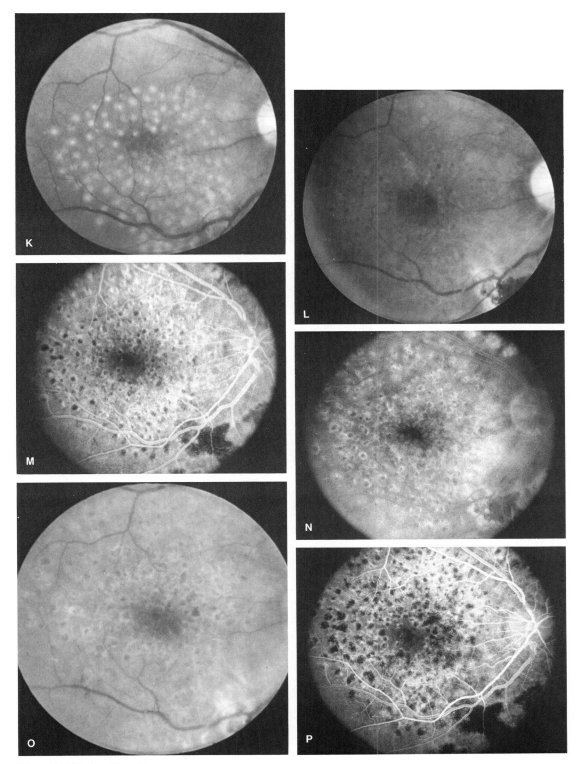

Figure 5–17 (continued)

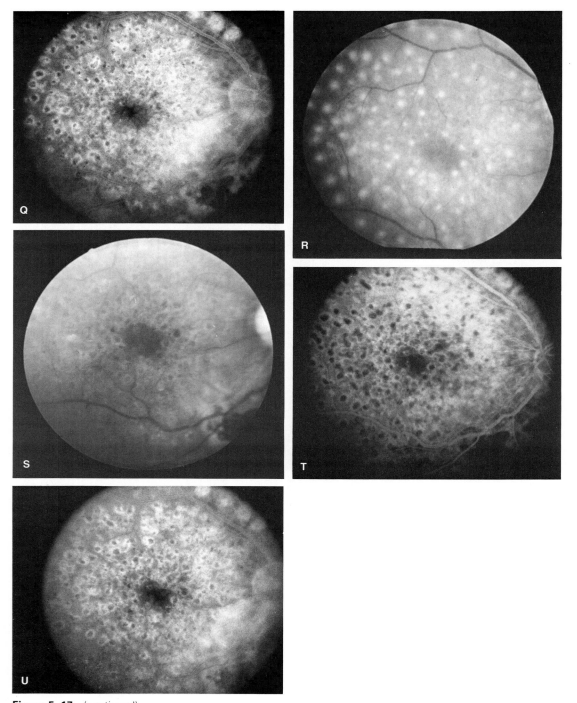

Figure 5–17 (continued)

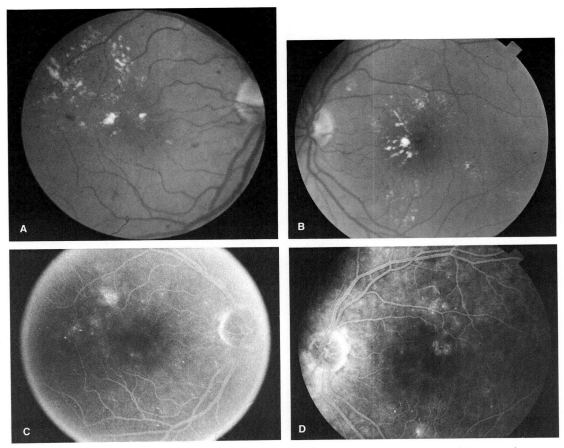

Figure 5–18 A 52-year-old white woman with type I insulin-dependent diabetes of 25-years duration (**A,B**) had an initial evaluation showing diffuse diabetic macular edema with (**C,D**) cystoid macular edema in both eyes. Initial visual acuity was 20/30 OD and 20/60 OS. (**E,F**) The right eye was treated with argon green and the left eye with krypton red modified grid laser photocoagulation. (**G–J**) Four months after the first treatment, central retinal thickening and cystoid macular edema persisted, and (**K,L**) both eyes received supplemental modified grid treatment. (**M,N**) Four months later, central retinal thickening still persisted in the right eye, and (**O**) a second supplemental modified grid treatment was given to the right eye. (**P–S**) One year after the initial treatment, both eyes showed that central retinal thickening and cystoid macular edema had resolved with visual acuity of 20/25. (**T,U**) One year after initial treatment vision was stable at 20/25, and (**V,W**) 5 years after the initial treatment vision remained stable at 20/25.

(continued)

angiography is indicated at this stage. Color fundus stereophotographs, however, may be helpful in documenting change, either progression or resolution, at the return visit.

We advise patients before treatment for diabetic macular edema that our goal is to maintain their current level of vision and to try to prevent further visual loss. We tell them that, although their vision may improve, that is not our intended goal. We also warn patients of the possibility of mild, but permanent, paracentral scotomata, especially following supplemental treatment, but that the long-term benefit of treatment outweighs this potential side effect (Figs. 5-17 and 5-18).

(continued on page 83)

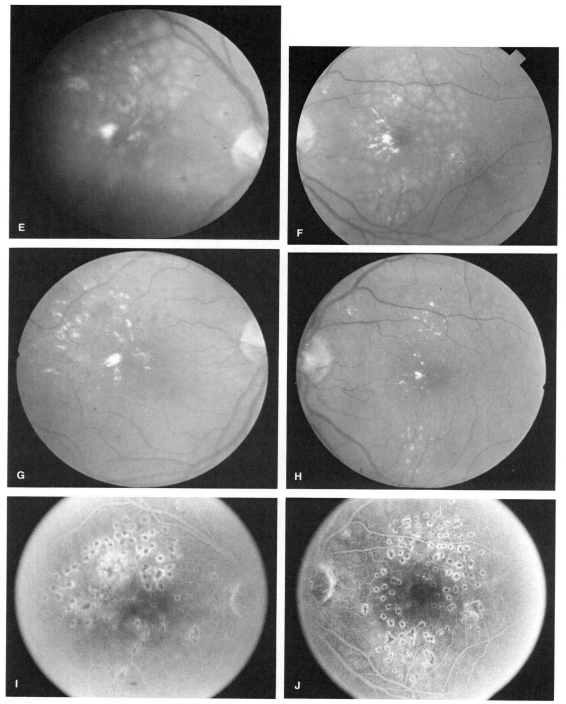

Figure 5–18   (continued)

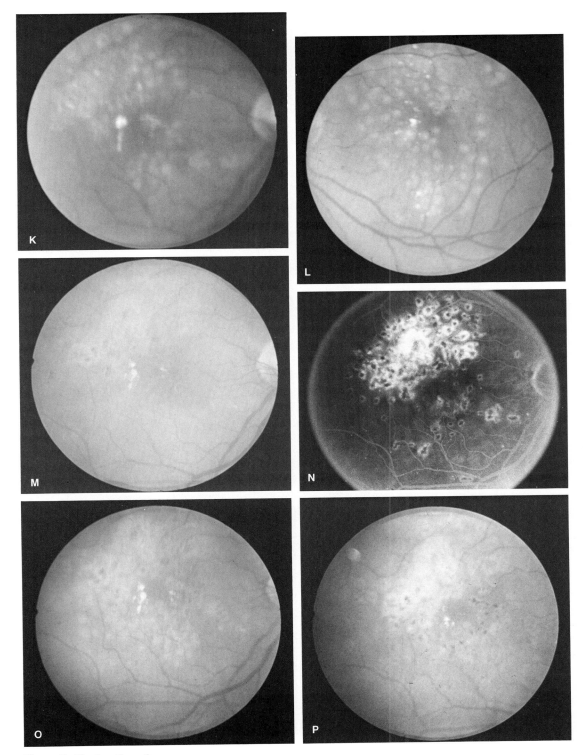

Figure 5–18 (continued)

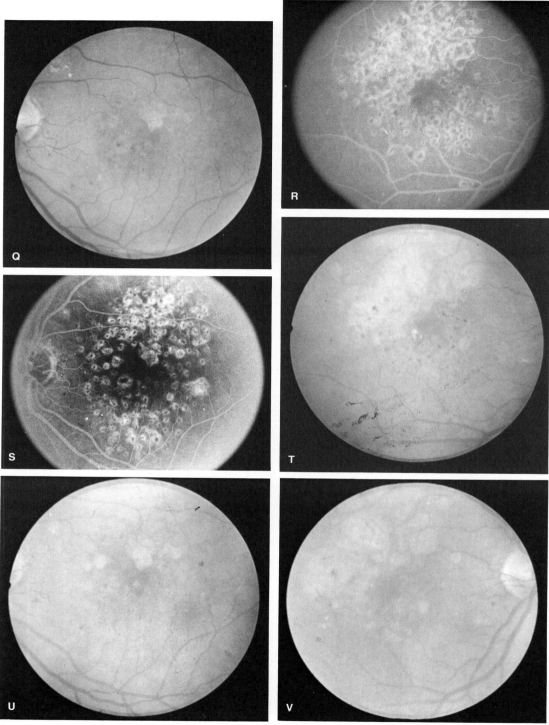

Figure 5–18 (continued)

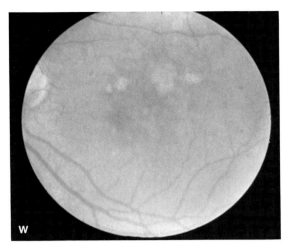

Figure 5–18 (continued)

References

1. Patz A, Schatz H, Berkow JE, et al. Macular edema: an overlooked complication of diabetic retinopathy. Trans Am Acad Ophthalmol Otolaryngol 1973; 77: 34–42.
2. McMeel JW, Trempe CL, Franks EB. Symposium: current status of photocoagulation of macular disease: diabetic maculopathy. Trans Am Acad Ophthalmol Otolaryngol 1977; 83:476–487.
3. Ferris FL, Patz A. Macular edema. A complication of diabetic retinopathy. Surv Ophthalmol 1984; 28:452–461.
4. Sigelman J. Diabetic macular edema in juvenile and adult-onset diabetes. Am J Ophthalmol 1980; 90:287–296.
5. Ferris FL, Podgor MJ, Davis MD. The Diabetic Retinopathy Study Research Group, Report No. 12. Macular edema in diabetic retinopathy study patients. Ophthalmology 1987; 94:754–760.
6. Klein R, Klein BEK, Moss SE, Davis MD, DeMets DL. The Wisconsin Epidemiologic Study of Diabetic Retinopathy. VI. Diabetic macular edema. Ophthalmology 1984; 91:1464–1474.
7. Klein R, Klein BEK, Moss SE, Davis MD, DeMets DL. The Wisconsin Epidemiologic Study of Diabetic Retinopathy. IX. Four-year incidence and progression of diabetic retinopathy when age at diagnosis is less than 30 years. Arch Ophthalmol 1989; 107:237–243.
8. Kohner EM. The evolution and natural history of diabetic retinopathy. Int Ophthalmol Clin 1978; 18 (4):1–16.
9. Aiello LM, Rand LI, Briones JC, Wafai MZ, Sebestyen JG. Diabetic retinopathy in Joslin Clinic patients with adult-onset diabetes. Ophthalmology 1981; 88:619–623.
10. Klein R, Klein BEK, Moss SE, DeMets DL, Kaufman I, Voss P. Prevalence of diabetes mellitus in Southern Wisconsin. Am J Epidemiol 1984; 119:54–61.
11. Klein R, Klein BEK, Moss SE. Visual impairment in diabetes. Ophthalmology 1984; 91:1–8.
12. Moss SE, Klein R, Klein BEK. The incidence of vision loss in a diabetic population. Ophthalmology 1988; 95:1340–1348.
13. Early Treatment Diabetic Retinopathy Study Research Group. ETDRS Report No. 1. Photocoagulation for diabetic macular edema. Arch Ophthalmol 1985; 103:1796–1806.
14. Early Treatment Diabetic Retinopathy Study Research Group. ETDRS Report No. 2. Treatment techniques and clinical guidelines for photocoagulation of diabetic macular edema. Ophthalmology 1987; 94:761–774.
15. Early Treatment Diabetic Retinopathy Study Research Group. ETDRS Report No. 4. Photocoagulation for diabetic macular edema. Int Ophthalmol Clin 1987; 27:265–272.
16. Blankenship GW. Diabetic macular edema and argon laser photocoagulation: a prospective randomized study. Ophthalmology 1979; 86:69–75.
17. British Multicentre Study Group. Photocoagulation for diabetic maculopathy. A randomized controlled clinical trial using the xenon arc. Diabetes 1983; 32:1010–1016.
18. Olk RJ. Modified grid argon (blue-green) laser photocoagulation for diffuse diabetic macular edema. Ophthalmology 1986; 93:938–950.
19. Olk RJ. Argon green (514 nm) versus krypton red (647 nm) modified grid laser photocoagulation for diffuse diabetic macular edema. Ophthalmology 1990; 97:1101–1113.
20. Kinyoun J, et al. Detection of diabetic macular edema: ophthalmology versus photography. Early Treatment Diabetic Retinopathy Study Report No. 5. Ophthalmology 1989; 96:746–751.
21. Early Treatment Diabetic Retinopathy Study Research Group. ETDRS Report No. 10. Grading diabetic retinopathy from stereoscopic color fundus photographs—an extension of the modified Airlie House classification. Ophthalmology 1991; 98:786–806.
22. Crues AF, Williams JC, Willan AR. Argon green and krypton red laser treatment of diabetic macular edema. Can J Ophthalmol 1988; 23:262–266.
23. Kayazawa F, DeJesus GT, Miyake K. Grid-pattern laser photocoagulation for diabetic diffuse macular edema (the Japanese experience). In: Gitter KA, Schatz H, Yannuzzi LA, et al., eds. Laser photocoagulation of retinal disease. San Francisco: Pacific Medical Press; 1988:65–68.
24. McDonald HR, Schatz H. Grid photocoagulation for diffuse macular edema. Retina 1985; 5:65–72.
25. Casswell AG, Canning CR, Gregor ZJ. Treatment of diffuse diabetic macular edema: a comparison be-

tween argon and krypton lasers. Eye 1990; 4:668–672.

26. Olk RJ. Argon-green vs krypton-red modified grid laser photocoagulation for diffuse diabetic macular edema. In: Gitter KA, Schatz H, Yannuzzi LA, et al., eds. Laser photocoagulation of retinal disease. San Francisco: Pacific Medical Press; 1988:75–81.

27. Lee CM, Olk RJ. Modified grid laser photocoagulation for diffuse diabetic macular edema: long-term visual results. Ophthalmology 1991; 98:1594–1602.

28. Clover GM. The effects of argon and krypton photocoagulation on the retina: implications for the inner and outer blood retinal barriers. In: Gitter KA, Schatz H, Yannuzzi LA, et al., eds. Laser photocoagulation of retinal disease. San Francisco: Pacific Medical Press; 1988:11–18.

29. Wallow IH. Repair of the pigment epithelial barrier following photocoagulation. Arch Ophthalmol 1984; 102:126–135.

30. Ansell PL, Marshall J. Laser-induced phagocytosis in the pigment epithelium of the Hunter dystrophic rat. Br J Ophthalmol 1976; 60:819–828.

31. Bresnick GH. Diabetic maculopathy: a critical review highlighting diffuse macular edema. Ophthalmology 1983; 90:1301–1317.

32. Welter J, Zuckerman R. The influence of the photoreceptor–RPE complex on the inner retina. An explanation for the beneficial effects of photocoagulation. Ophthalmology 1980; 87:1133–1139.

33. Striph GG, Hart WM, Olk RJ. Modified grid laser photocoagulation for diabetic macular edema. The effect on the central visual field. Ophthalmology 1988; 95:1673–1679.

34. Mainster MA. Wavelength selection in macular photocoagulation: tissue optics, thermal effects, and laser systems. Ophthalmology 1986; 93:952–958.

35. Early Treatment Diabetic Retinopathy Study Research Group. ETDRS Report No. 9. Early photocoagulation for diabetic retinopathy. Ophthalmology 1991; 98:766–785.

Diabetic Retinopathy: Practical Management, by
R. Joseph Olk and Carol M. Lee. J.B. Lippincott Company, Philadelphia © 1993.

CHAPTER · 6

Management of Proliferative Diabetic Retinopathy

HIGH-RISK PROLIFERATIVE RETINOPATHY

Epidemiology

Diabetes is the leading cause of blindness in Americans aged 25 to 74 years,[1] blindness being the final adverse sequela of proliferative retinopathy. The Wisconsin Epidemiologic Study of Diabetic Retinopathy (WESDR) showed that the prevalence of proliferative retinopathy is directly related to the duration of the disease, with 0% seen in younger-onset insulin-dependent patients with fewer than 5 years of diabetes, to 4% in patients with 9 to 10 years of diabetes, to 26% in patients with diabetes of 15 to 16 years, and 56% in patients with diabetes of 20 or more years[2] (Figs. 6-1 and 6-2). This correlation with duration is also present in older-onset individuals, both insulin and non–insulin-dependent; however, approximately 3% to 4% of all older-onset patients with diabetes of 4 years or less had evidence of proliferative retinopathy. After at least 15 years of diabetes, 20% of older-onset insulin-dependent individuals, but only 4% of older-onset non–insulin-dependent individuals, had evidence of proliferative retinopathy.[3]

Despite these figures on the prevalence of proliferative disease and the unequivocal benefit of treatment for certain levels of retinopathy, the WESDR revealed another alarming statistic: 26% of 909 younger-onset and 36% of 1370 older-onset diabetic patients had never had an ophthalmologic examination.[4] Eleven percent of younger-onset and 7% of older-onset diabetic patients who had high-risk retinopathy when entered into the WESDR study either had never been seen by an ophthalmologist or had not been seen by any ophthalmologist in more than 2 years.[4] In addition, this study examined the prevalence of photocoagulation in a population-based fashion and found that 55% of eyes seen with high-risk retinopathy when entered into another arm of the WESDR had not been treated with photocoagulation.[5] Even more impressive is the incidence report on photocoagulation during 4 years follow-up: 42% of younger-onset eyes with high-risk retinopathy had not been treated at entry into this study, but 34% still had yet to receive photocoagulation after 4 years.[6] Of older-onset diabetics with high-risk retinopathy 69% and 58% had never received photocoagulation at 1 and 4 years, respectively. Thus the rate of appropriate detection, management, treatment,

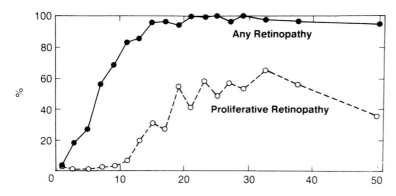

Figure 6–1 Frequency of retinopathy or proliferative retinopathy by duration of diabetes (in years) in persons taking insulin who had a diagnosis of diabetes before 30 years of age and who participated in the Wisconsin Epidemiologic Study of Diabetic Retinopathy, 1980–1982. (From Klein R, et al. The Wisconsin Epidemiologic Study of Diabetic Retinopathy. II. Prevalence and risk of diabetic retinopathy when age at diagnosis is less than 30 years. Arch Ophthalmol 1984; 102:520–526.)

and follow-up was inadequate, especially given the advances of the last two decades in the prevention of severe visual loss owing to diabetes. This disparity is presently being addressed by the Diabetes 2000 project to reduce the number of cases of preventable blindness caused by diabetes.

Indication for Treatment

The first step in the management of the diabetic eye is the identification of significant retinopathy. A careful examination of the entire retina, concentrating especially on the posterior pole and midperiphery, looking for evidence of proliferative disease, is crucial. A complete 360° peripheral examination aided by scleral depression should be performed. Careful examination of the iris surface and pupillary margin using slit-lamp biomicroscopy and magnification should be performed, looking for fine iris neovascularization. The angle geome-

try of each diabetic eye should be examined with gonioscopy, using a mirrored contact lens, such as the Zeiss lens or four-mirror Goldmann lens. The latter, however, if used with a viscous contact lens solution may impair the quality of fluorescein angiography or fundus photography if needed later in the examination.

The Diabetic Retinopathy Study (DRS) has described proliferative retinopathy in terms of retinopathy risk factors.[7–11] As discussed in Chapter 3, these are defined by

1. The *presence* of new vessels
2. The *location* of new vessels, either on the disc or within one disc diameter of the optic disc (NVD) or elsewhere on the retina (NVE)
3. The *severity* of new vessels
4. The presence of preretinal or vitreous *hemorrhage.*

In considering the severity of new vessels, if both NVD and NVE were present, only the se-

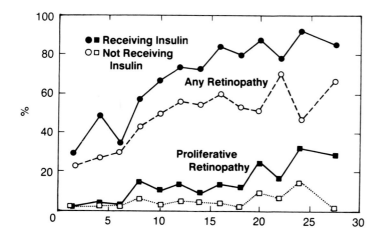

Figure 6–2 Frequency of retinopathy or proliferative retinopathy by duration of diabetes (in years) in persons receiving (*black circles* or *black squares*) or not receiving (*white circles* or *white squares*) insulin who had a diagnosis of diabetes at or after age 30. (From Klein R, et al. The Wisconsin Epidemiologic Study of Diabetic Retinopathy. III. Prevalence and risk of diabetic retinopathy when age at diagnosis is 30 or more years. Arch Ophthalmol 1984; 102:527–532.)

verity of the disc vessels was counted, since the DRS showed that the presence of moderate or severe NVE did not further increase the risk for severe visual loss when compared with NVD alone. For NVD, NVD had to be greater than or equal to standard photograph 10A or one-third or one-fourth disc area in size. For NVE, NVE had to be greater or equal to one-half disc area in at least one photographic field. The combination of any three of the above four retinopathy risk factors is considered to place an eye at high risk for severe visual loss. These high-risk eyes unequivocally benefit from panretinal photocoagulation, which in the DRS reduced the rate of severe visual loss by one-half, from 44% of control eyes to approximately 20% of treated eyes at 4-years follow-up.

Three clinically recognizable situations are characteristic of high-risk retinopathy. These are

1. Moderate-to-severe NVD (greater than or equal to standard photograph 10A), with or without preretinal or vitreous hemorrhage
2. Less extensive NVD with preretinal or vitreous hemorrhage
3. Moderate-to-severe NVE (greater than one-half disc area) with preretinal or vitreous hemorrhage.

Immediate photocoagulation is indicated when these clinical high-risk conditions exist or when any combination of retinopathy risk factors equals three—in other words, high-risk retinopathy.

Proliferative retinopathy should be detected clinically, on a dilated fundus examination. For purposes of documentation and to follow the response to photocoagulation, color stereophotographs may be obtained using the standard "seven stereo fields"; expanded 60°-wide field photographs may provide more complete photographic documentation than overlapping 30° photographs.[12]

In general, we do not routinely order fluorescein angiography before treatment, as proliferative changes should be recognized on the clinical examination. In cases of questionable neovascularization, for instance, subtle early NVE versus intraretinal microvascular abnormalities (IRMA), fluorescein angiography may

be helpful in determining between the two. This distinction may be difficult to make, however, as IRMA may also leak. Only if there is difficulty in differentiating between neovascularization or IRMA or if preretinal or vitreous hemorrhage exists, the source of which is not clinically evident, is fluorescein angiography obtained. In the latter situation, localization of flat NVE through the preretinal or vitreous hemorrhage may be possible with fluorescein angiography or angioscopy.

Anterior neovascularization or rubeosis is another indication for immediate treatment. This, too, should be detectable on clinical examination. Once the decision to treat has been made, photocoagulation should be scheduled promptly; in the case of rubeosis, urgent treatment is especially important.[13–15]

Practical Guidelines for Initial Treatment

The original protocols of the DRS employed either argon blue-green or xenon arc photocoagulation. It was found that both a greater initial loss of visual acuity and a greater constriction of the peripheral visual field could be attributed to the xenon group. No statistical difference in visual outcome could be delineated between argon blue-green or xenon arc photocoagulation by the DRS or other comparative studies[16,17] (Fig. 6-3).

In the Early Treatment Diabetic Retinopathy Study (ETDRS), argon green became available in December 1982, and because the green wavelength theoretically precludes the additional uptake of blue wavelength by the macular xanthophyll,[18] the ETDRS[19] effected a protocol change in its study guidelines and began to use the argon green wavelength for all protocols involving panretinal photocoagulation, in addition to the argon blue-green wavelength. The use of krypton red was allowed when significant cataract or vitreous hemorrhage precluded adequate uptake or treatment by the argon modality.

We currently perform photocoagulation for proliferative retinopathy with the argon green modality and save the krypton red wavelength for eyes with vitreous hemorrhage or advanced

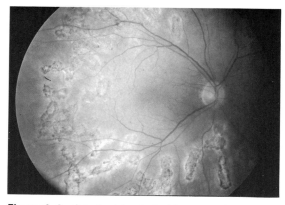

Figure 6–3 A patient treated with xenon photocoagulation for proliferative diabetic retinopathy, with complete regression of her retinopathy. Note the confluent scars typical of xenon treatment.

cataract. Although krypton red theoretically produces less damage to the nerve fiber layer and inner retina,[18] studies by Olk[20] and others[21,22] found no comparative difference in the outcome of eyes treated for diabetic macular edema with argon green, compared with krypton red. Schulenberg and associates[23] and Blankenship[24] also found no significant difference between argon blue-green and krypton red in either efficacy or side effects relative to treatment of proliferative diabetic retinopathy.[23,24] The recently completed Krypton Argon Regression of Neovascularization Study (KARNS) concluded that argon blue-green laser photocoagulation was equally as effective as krypton red in the treatment of high-risk proliferative retinopathy, looking specifically at the regression of neovascularization of the disc as defined by the DRS.[25,26] The decision as to which wavelength to choose should be based on other pertinent clinical findings, such as the presence of vitreous hemorrhage, given that the argon and krypton wavelengths appear to be of equal benefit in the management of proliferative disease.

A panfunduscopic lens or similar wide-angle lens, such as the Rodenstock or Volk Quadraspheric lens, is applied to the eye, and argon green is used unless significant cataract or other media opacity, such as vitreous hemorrhage, exists. The entire posterior pole and midperiphery is visible with one field of view, so that both the fovea and the disc are readily visualized. Remember that the view through a panfunduscopic lens is both inverted and reversed. In other words, the view through the Rodenstock lens of a right fundus would place the disc in the temporal half of the field of view; a point along the inferior half of the retina would be seen in the superior field of view.

The retinal surface is carefully focused. Focusing through a panfunduscopic lens is most easily accomplished initially with the rays of light from the slit-lamp directed perpendicular to the surface of the lens. The rays are then directed more tangentially to avoid the reflections from the surface of the lens. Once the retinal surface is visualized and the location of the landmarks of the retina are easily recognized by the laser surgeon, the aiming beam is set at the lowest intensity, still allowing adequate visualization of the aiming beam. We try to perform all panretinal scatter treatments with either the 500- or 400-μm spot size with 0.1- to 0.2-second duration. The Rodenstock lens allows a magnification effect, giving an actual burn of 668 μm[27] to 810 μm[28] for a burn set at 500 μm; in comparison, the Goldmann lens gives a diameter approximately equivalent to the spot setting.[28] It is sometimes difficult to aim and laser the 500-μm spot size when a significant cataract is present. Reducing the spot size, then, to 400 μm will make it easier to produce an adequate burn. Also, when decreasing the spot size, to maintain an equivalent burn, the power of the laser burn must generally be decreased by an equivalent proportion. In addition, although the rotating cylinder of marked spot sizes may not have present an indentation or "click" for 400 μm, setting the rotating cylinder a distance of two-thirds away from the setting of 200 μm will approximate the setting for a 400-μm spot size.

Typically, we start at approximately 200 mW of power, slowly increasing the power in 25 to 50-mW increments to achieve a moderately white burn. The endpoint here is a darker spot than in macular treatments and usually requires a higher power setting in eyes with lighter fundi. Increasing the duration will also help if it is difficult to obtain adequate laser burns in conditions of hypopigmentation, serous detachment, or retinal edema.

We first delineate the temporal foveal border of the panretinal photocoagulation with three to four rows of laser burns placed in an arcuate fashion at least two disc diameters from the fovea; these barrier rows aid in the prevention of inadvertent treatment of the fovea (Fig. 6-4). Throughout the course of treatment, the optic disc and fovea are repeatedly visualized and, when treating in the midperiphery, frequent scans of the posterior pole remind the laser surgeon of the geography of the retina. Laser spots are placed approximately one burn width apart. Serial repeat treatment or pretreatment of laser burns with differing spot sizes is not recommended. For instance, we do not first treat with 200-μm spots and then retreat over that with a larger-spot size. In panretinal photocoagulation, the individual peripheral microaneurysms are not treated focally.

In general, we divide a full-scatter panretinal photocoagulation into two sessions. First, the inferior one-half of the retina is treated with 800 to 1000 burns (Fig. 6-5). Laser burns are brought up to one disc diameter from the optic disc; NVD is not treated directly. We prefer to treat the inferior one-half of the retina first so that if significant vitreous hemorrhage were to occur between the two sessions, the hemorrhage would then settle more inferiorly owing to gravity, allowing treatment to the superior portion of the retina (Fig. 6-6).

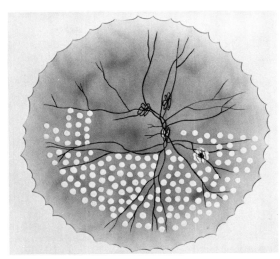

Figure 6–5 First session of panretinal photocoagulation: The inferior half of the retina is then treated with 500-μm spot size burns at approximately one-burn width apart for 800 to 1000 laser burns. Confluent local treatment is applied to the retina underlying flat surface NVE.

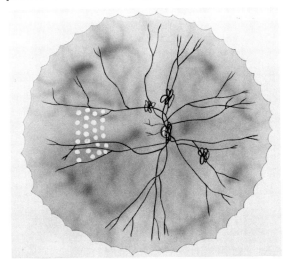

Figure 6–4 First session of panretinal photocoagulation: Barrier row for panretinal photocoagulation placing three to four rows of 500-μm spots at least two disc diameters from the center of the macula is helpful in delineating the macular border of treatment.

Local treatment of the retina underlying flat surface NVE that is smaller than two disc areas is performed with slightly overlapping confluent 500-μm moderate white burns. The NVE is treated in this focal fashion as long as it is at least one disc diameter from the optic disc and two disc diameters or more from the center of the fovea temporally and generally outside the superotemporal and inferotemporal arcades. We do not attempt to directly close the new retinal vessels by the laser treatment because this may be associated with vitreous hemorrhage. Instead, we aim at the retinal tissue underlying the flat surface NVE; the whitening seen is that of the retina and not of the NVE itself. We do not treat elevated NVE nor any NVD directly (Fig. 6-7).

For the second session, patients are scheduled to return within 2 to 3 weeks for completion of the panretinal photocoagulation. The superior one-half of the retina is then treated with scatter panretinal and focal ablation of NVE with another series of 800 to 1000 500-μm spots (Fig. 6-8). We specifically avoid application of treatment to major vessels or chorioretinal scars, areas of preretinal blood, and areas of elevated neovascularization. Changes

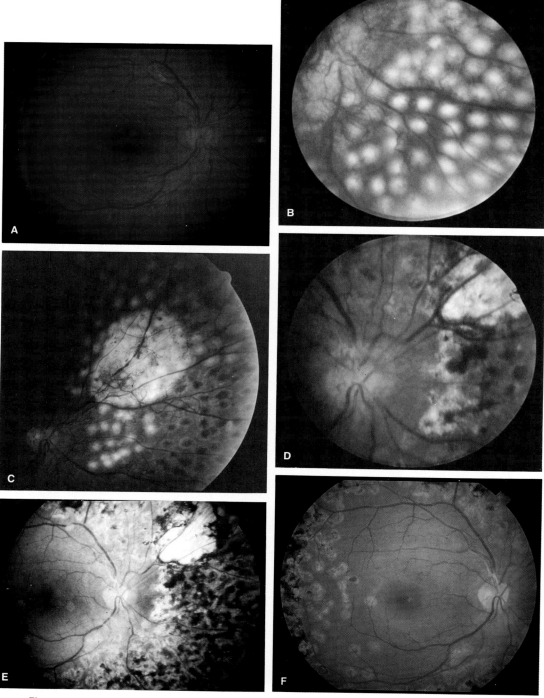

Figure 6–6 (**A**) A 16-year-old white girl presented with high-risk retinopathy. (**B**) Panretinal photocoagulation treatment to the inferior one-half of the retina was performed. Note that the spots are placed approximately one spot size apart with the goal of a moderate white burn. The laser spots were brought up to one disc diameter of the optic nerve head. (**C**) Two weeks later the superior one-half of the retina was treated. The surface NVE was treated with confluent photocoagulation burns. (**D**) At 6 months, her NVD was regressing and (**E**) at 1 year and (**F**) 2 years after panretinal photocoagulation she had no evidence of recurrent proliferative disease.

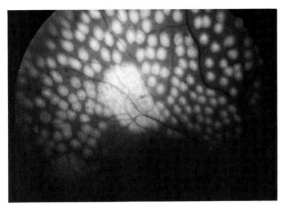

Figure 6–7 If NVE is flat along the retinal surface, confluent ablation can be performed using overlapping laser photocoagulation burns, with the goal of a white lesion. Confluent ablation should not be performed if the NVE is elevated. The NVD should never be directly ablated.

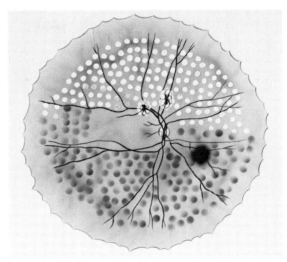

Figure 6–8 Second session of panretinal photocoagulation: The superior half of the retina is treated at 2 to 3 weeks after the initial session, again with 500-μm spot size burns at approximately one-burn width apart for 800 to 1000 laser burns. Confluent local treatment is applied to the retina underlying flat surface NVE.

consistent with vascular occlusive retinopathy can be seen following direct treatment of large retinal vessels (Figs. 6-9 through 6-11). Although we are not aware of any specific studies documenting the exacerbation of tractional elements with laser photocoagulation over the natural course of the disease, it is our clinical practice to avoid direct treatment of tractionally elevated fibrovascular proliferation.

We treat up to the anterior margin of the equator, using both a panfunduscopic lens and,

if necessary, a three-mirror Goldmann lens. If switching between the two lenses, the appropriate orientation and geography of the retina must always be maintained to avoid inadvertent macular treatment. The power setting of the laser should also be lowered when switch-

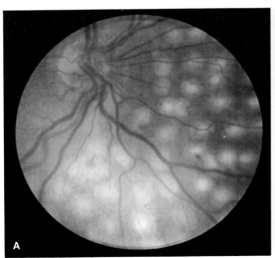
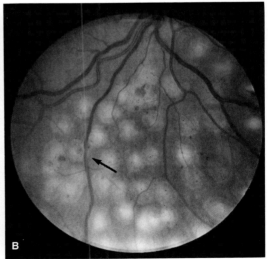

Figure 6–9 An example of panretinal treatment technique. (**A**) Note that the spots are approximately one burn apart and one disc diameter from the optic nerve head. These laser spots were placed with a Rodenstock lens. (**B**) Note the avoidance of the major vessels, and in an area where the laser burn touched the vessel, there is slight constriction (*inferiorly*) in **B**.

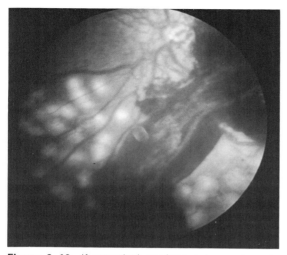

Figure 6–10 If preretinal or vitreous hemorrhage is seen, the visible retina should be treated, avoiding direct treatment of the blood. In this eye, krypton red laser photocoagulation was used because of the media opacity created by the scattered vitreous hemorrhage.

ing from the panfunduscopic to the Goldmann lens if maintaining the same spot size.

We generally perform panretinal photocoagulation using a retrobulbar or peribulbar anesthetic with a 50:50 mixture of 2% lidocaine and 0.75% bupivacaine with hyaluronidase for krypton treatments. If both macular and panretinal photocoagulation is given for combined diabetic macular edema and proliferative disease, retrobulbar anesthetic may also be employed (see Chapter 10, Special Cases). However, because of the concurrent akinesia that accompanies the analgesia, peripheral treatment is sometimes difficult to perform, as the patient will be unable to move his or her eyes to aid with the use of the lens.

When topical anesthesia is employed, patients generally tolerate panretinal photocoagulation with minimal discomfort; however, some patients are particularly sensitive to treatment without an anesthetic in the region

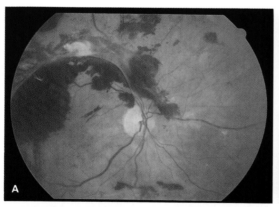

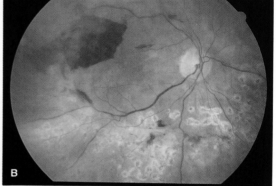

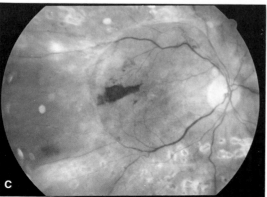

Figure 6–11 A patient presented with (**A**) proliferative diabetic retinopathy, with preretinal and vitreous hemorrhage and traction from fibrous proliferation along the superotemporal arcades. The patient received two sessions of panretinal photocoagulation, avoiding direct treatment of the fibrous tissue and hemorrhage. (**B**) Three months later there was resorption of hemorrhage with no new evidence of reproliferation. No additional treatment was given. Seven months later, visual acuity was 20/60 and (**C**) fundus examination showed involuted proliferative disease and a good panretinal photocoagulation pattern, with no evidence of recurrent proliferative disease and minimal residual preretinal hemorrhage.

of the long ciliary nerves. We have found that lowering the spot size with the necessary lowering of the power to achieve the same intensity burn will relieve the pain. If the spot size is lowered, more total laser burns need to be placed to treat the same area of retina. This usually allows completion of the session, without the need for a retrobulbar or peribulbar anesthetic.

Postoperatively, patients are given a mild oral nonprescription analgesic, such as acetaminophen. Patients are instructed to avoid heavy lifting, bending from the waist, or excessive straining if significant new vessels or preretinal or vitreous hemorrhage was noted. If vitreous hemorrhage is present, patients are also instructed to sleep with their head elevated by two to three pillows. Patients are advised that there should be minimal to no discomfort following laser therapy; they are told to return immediately if severe pain occurs because this could herald angle closure caused by choroidal effusion and anterior ciliary body rotation (see Chapter 9, Complications and Side Effects of Treatment). We give topical steroids and cycloplegics for 1 week following a session of panretinal photocoagulation. In our experience, this has minimized the iritis and synechiae formation that can occur after panretinal laser treatment. The first follow-up appointment is scheduled for 6 to 8 weeks following completion of the initial panretinal photocoagulation (Fig. 6-12).

The optimal number of photocoagulation burns needed to initiate and cause regression of the new vessels is unknown.[24–27] Complete initial panretinal photocoagulation is generally considered from 1500 to 2000 spots. The order of treatment and the number of sessions—single versus multiple—have also been studied.[29–33] Relative to the regression of proliferative retinopathy, the increase in tractional detachment, or the increase in vitreous hemorrhage, there appears to be no significant difference between panretinal photocoagulation delivered in one session, versus two or more sessions.[27] However, the adverse side effects of choroidal effusion, exudative retinal detachment, and angle closure[29,33] may be less frequent if the panretinal treatment is performed

in multiple sessions. For patients who find it a great hardship to return for treatment in a timely fashion or if compliance is a question, single-session treatment may be advised.

If very severe proliferative disease is being treated, we will often initially plan for more extensive treatment, with a plan of 2000 to 3000 burns in two to four divided sessions. In general, however, we do not recommend placing more than 1000 to 1200 burns at any given session, because the more burns placed, the higher the likelihood of adverse sequelae. The specific pattern of treatment is up to the individual surgeon.

The importance of the midperipheral retinal vasculature and occlusions was demonstrated by Shimuzi and associates,[34] and it is felt that these midperipheral ischemic changes may cause the development of neovascularization, both on the disc and elsewhere.[34–37] As long as the midperipheral retinal areas are completely treated, it probably makes no difference whether the inferior retina was treated before the superior retina or whether the nasal retina was treated before the temporal retina. We are also unsure of exactly how laser photocoagulation works to aid in the regression of neovascularization. As discussed in Chapter 5, multiple theories, ranging from destruction of the ischemic retina, thereby decreasing the angiogenic stimulus; improved oxygenation of the remaining retina; or enhanced retinal pigment epithelium (RPE) function, have been postulated.

Indication for Supplemental Treatment

Regression of neovascularization is obviously the goal of photocoagulation, but this may not be complete. In fact, regression is usually not complete, as seen in the DRS[8,11,38] and numerous other reports.[16,29–32,39,40] In the DRS, complete regression of NVD in eyes with high-risk retinopathy at 1-year follow-up was seen in only 21% of eyes treated with panretinal photocoagulation. Eyes will often move from high-risk categories, with three or four retinopathy risk factors, to low-risk categories, with residual milder neovascularization. In Doft and

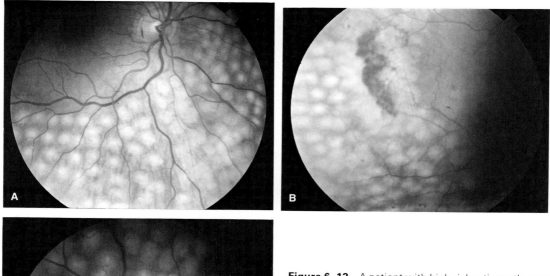

Figure 6–12 A patient with high-risk retinopathy was treated with panretinal photocoagulation in two sessions. (**A**) The inferior one-half of the retina is shown with (**B**) confluent ablation of the surface NVE, followed 2 weeks later (**C**) by completion of the panretinal photocoagulation to the superior one-half of the retina. Note that the laser photocoagulation spots are brought usually up to one disc diameter from the edge of the optic nerve, and the spots are usually placed outside the inferotemporal and superotemporal arcades and (**B**) are no closer than two disc diameters from the temporal edge of the foveal avascular zone.

Blankenship's study, 72% of eyes treated for high-risk retinopathy improved, with a drop to non–high-risk categories by 3 weeks following completion of panretinal photocoagulation of 1200 spots of 500-μm size.[31] By 6 months, 72% of these eyes continued to remain at less than high-risk. Of these eyes, 42% had no evidence of proliferative disease, whereas 31% had some evidence of mild proliferative disease, but less than high risk.[31] High-risk features persisted at 6-month follow-up in nearly two-thirds of the original 28% of eyes that did not demonstrate an early favorable response to treatment. In another recent study by Vander and colleagues,[41] the favorable early response of eyes with high-risk retinopathy to photocoagulation at 3 months was carried out for up to 4 years of follow-up, supported by both better visual acuity and lack of recurrent high-risk retinopathy. This initial favorable response to treatment was seen by 3 months.

The response to treatment is often noted early in follow-up, within the first 6 to 8 weeks. In those eyes that either show no or minimal improvement in their clinical picture, supplemental photocoagulation is recommended.[19,30,39] Other indications for supplemental treatment include retinopathy that appears to be progressing, new NVD, new rubeosis, new vitreous or preretinal hemorrhage, and the comparative extent and location of previous photocoagulation.[19] Supplemental or "fill-in" treatment should be performed if there are other clinical indications or if the previous pattern of treatment is scanty, incomplete, or has large skip areas. In a study by Vine, high-risk eyes were

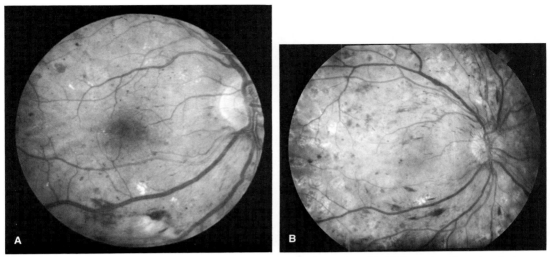

Figure 6–13 A patient presented with (**A**) high-risk retinopathy with NVD greater than standard photograph 10A. (**B**) Two months after completion of his initial panretinal photocoagulation NVD had increased. This is an indication for supplemental panretinal photocoagulation.

treated with additional scatter photocoagulation if they showed minimal to no favorable response at 2 months' follow-up to an initial scatter panretinal treatment of 3000 burns placed in three sessions.[39] Focal ablation to the retina underlying flat neovascularization was not performed in this study. Additional treatment caused a favorable response, with a reduction in risk factors to a low-risk category in 50% of eyes[39] (Figs. 6-13 through 6-15).

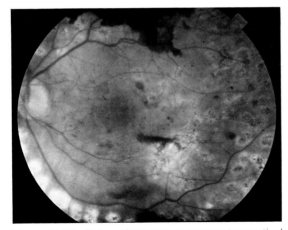

Figure 6–14 This patient was status post-panretinal photocoagulation for high-risk retinopathy and presented with new preretinal hemorrhage from NVE. This is an indication for supplemental treatment.

It should also be noted that the DRS did not reveal any significant association between persistence of neovascularization or retinopathy risk factors and severe visual loss. Depending on the individual clinical situation, supplemental treatment may not be necessary. If a patient shows reasonable regression of his or her initially florid retinopathy with fine residual loops of NVD, an immediate supplemental treatment may not be needed, provided that adequate treatment already exists and that good follow-up can be maintained (Figs. 6-16 and 6-17). Here fundus photographs of the optic disc can be helpful to compare future findings looking for progression or regression of the NVD. Additional panretinal photocoagulation may also be given more conservatively following a complete posterior detachment, since vitreoretinal tractional elements may no longer be affected. Since the posterior hyaloid is now completely detached, further progression of the new vessels will theoretically not be accompanied by additional vitreoretinal traction.

Practical Guidelines for Supplemental Treatment

If a patient shows minimal to no regression of his retinopathy or has any of the previously de-

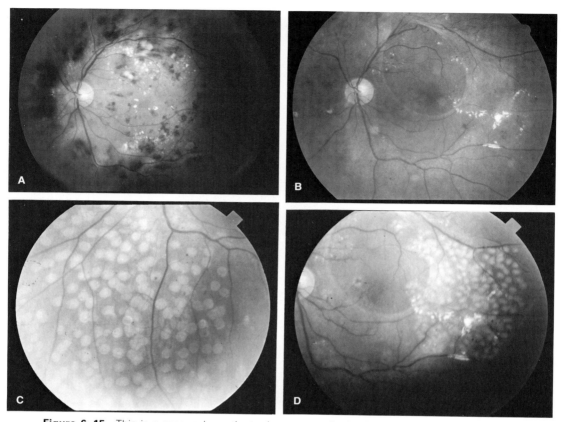

Figure 6–15 This is a monocular patient who presented with (**A**) very severe nonproliferative diabetic retinopathy with four-quadrants of severe retinal hemorrhage and prominent venous beading, especially superotemporally and failed to return for follow-up. (**B**) Four years later he returned with extensive fibrosis and numerous zones of NVE. Vitreous hemorrhage (not shown) was also present. Note the central opening through the posterior hyaloid face and its attachment along the superotemporal arcade. He underwent multiple sessions of panretinal photocoagulation for a total of 3000 burns over the next 6 weeks. (**C**) The first session involved panretinal photocoagulation to the inferior one-half of the retina, and (**D**) grid treatment applied to areas of retinal thickening and nonperfusion temporal to the macula. In the second panretinal photocoagulation session, (**E**) the temporal areas were treated, and (**F**) in the third session the treatment to the superior half of the retina was completed. (**G,H**) One month later, additional panretinal photocoagulation was given to completely fill in all areas of untreated retina. Because this patient was monocular and had a history of noncompliance, aggressive panretinal photocoagulation was applied over a relatively short period. Note that this patient demonstrated significant epiretinal fibrosis, and direct treatment of the fibrous tissue was avoided.

(continued)

scribed indications for supplemental treatment at the 6- to 8-week follow-up visit, supplemental panretinal photocoagulation is recommended. When supplemental treatment is given, settings similar to those used in the original treatment are recommended, filling in the spaces of untreated retina between the older photocoagulation scars. We give approximately 1000 burns of 500-μm spot size at the supplemental session and at each following

one, if necessary (Fig. 6-18). We extend the treatment anteriorly beyond the equator, with 500-μm spots and closer in toward the posterior pole, sometimes with one to two rows of treatment just within the arcade at 200-μm spot size. Alternatively, if residual or new surface neovascularization is located within the arcades, but at least one disc diameter from the center of the macula, we will treat the underlying retina with confluent overlapping 200-

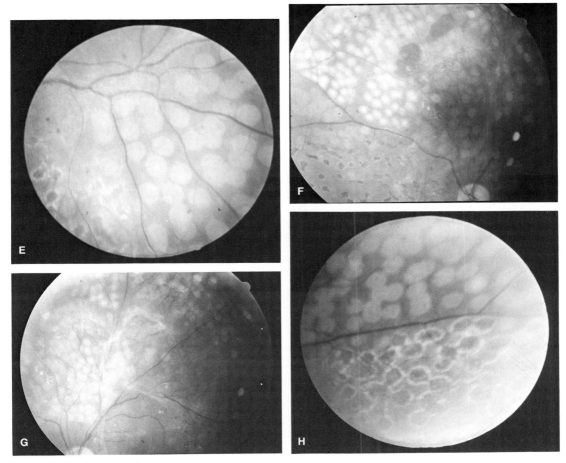

Figure 6–15 (continued)

μm burns. The temporal edge of the initial treatment located two disc diameters from the fovea often has marked capillary abnormalities—this area should be carefully retreated during supplemental sessions.

In circumstances under which extensive photocoagulation has already been placed, retreatment over previous treatment scars is sometimes necessary. In this latter situation, retinal tissue may be atrophied to the point that inadvertent rupture of Bruch's membrane may occur, with subsequent iatrogenic chorioretinal neovascularization. To avoid this complication, lighter intensity burns of longer duration using the argon wavelength are recommended if treatment over previous burns is necessary. This is especially true if earlier focal treatment of peripheral NVE has not caused regression, and repeat treatment is necessary to the underlying retina (Fig. 6-19).

Conversely, anterior cryotreatment or indirect laser photocoagulation with scleral indentation of the peripheral retina can be employed to treat previously untreated retina anterior to the equator, which might not be easily reached by the slit-lamp delivery system. This additional confluent treatment will usually produce irreversible peripheral visual field defects.

Once stabilization of the retinopathy is noted, patients are then seen at 3- to 4-month intervals. Panretinal photocoagulation is not indicated in eyes with end-stage fibroproliferative disease, when the originally perfused neovascular tissue is replaced by avascular

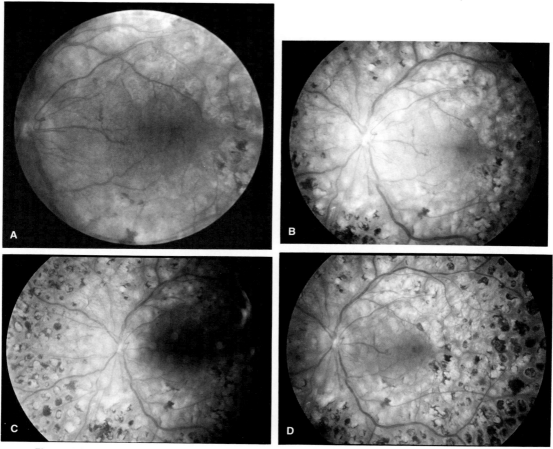

Figure 6–16 A 36-year-old man presented who had received panretinal photocoagulation and supplemental panretinal photocoagulation elsewhere for high-risk retinopathy. The patient demonstrated substantial regression of pretreatment of his NVD. However, (**A**) residual NVD was noted. (**B**) At 4 months, (**C**) 1 year, and (**D**) 2 years after presentation the residual NVD was unchanged. Because this patient showed no increase in his NVD or no episodes of new preretinal or vitreous hemorrhage, he did not require any supplemental treatment. If either new areas of NVE or increase in his NVD, or new preretinal or vitreous hemorrhage should be noted, supplemental treatment would then be advised.

gliotic tissue.[42] Other signs of this "burnt-out" picture include a pale optic disc, attenuated vessels, and a generally "featureless" retina.

CRYOTHERAPY

Cryotherapy is an important adjunct in the treatment of proliferative retinopathy.[43–47] If vitreous hemorrhage or significant cataract precludes an adequate view of the retina

through the slit-lamp system, cryotherapy has been shown to be efficacious in reducing retinopathy, although no large-scale national or case-controlled studies have been reported (Fig. 6-20).

Peripheral transconjunctival cryoapplications are performed only under a retrobulbar or peribulbar anesthetic. Typically 36 cryotherapy applications are given with two applications placed at each clock hour and one application at each half-hour between the ora serrata and the equator.[47] If this is supplemental treatment, we bring the cryoapplication up

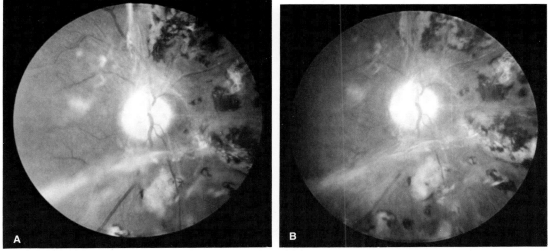

Figure 6–17 This eye is status post-panretinal photocoagulation for proliferative disease. There is fibrosis, and a tractional component nasally off the disc. (**A**) There is no evidence of active proliferative disease or bleeding, and this patient was followed every 4 to 6 months for the next 5 years. (**B**) No change was noted in his fibrous component, and no additional laser treatment was given.

to the edge of the previous photocoagulation scars under direct visualization (Fig. 6-21). With direct visualization through the indirect ophthalmoscope, the endpoint is retinal whitening, which generally takes from 4 to 8 seconds and is achieved at temperatures of −60°C to −80°C.[46] If no retina can be observed, for instance, owing to significant media hemorrhage, cryoapplications are held at −60°C for 3 to 4 seconds at 11 to 14 mm from the limbus, if the conjunctiva is intact.[43,47] (Figs. 6-22 and 6-23).

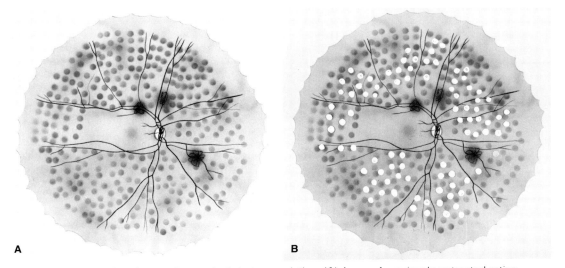

Figure 6–18 Supplemental panretinal photocoagulation. (**A**) Areas of previously untreated retina are now treated (**B**) with 500-μm spot size laser burns. We try to fill in the areas between spots, but occasionally treat over previous laser burns or treat over previously treated surface NVE. The retina underlying new zones of flat surface NVE are treated with confluent laser photocoagulation burns.

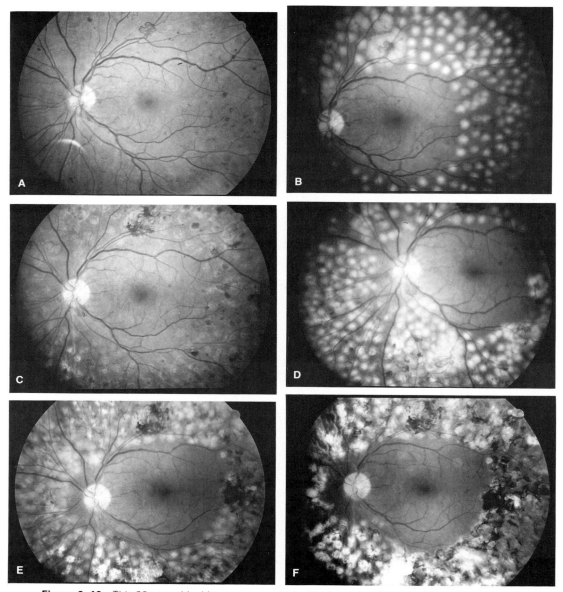

Figure 6–19 This 30-year-old white man presented with high-risk retinopathy (**A**) and was treated with PRP in two sessions. (**B**) The central zone was treated first, followed 2 weeks later by treatment of the peripheral zone. (**C**) Three months later he had persistent NVD, which had increased since presentation, and (**D**) he received supplemental panretinal photocoagulation. Note that the surface NVE is confluently treated. The NVD is not treated directly. He received another supplemental panretinal photocoagulation for (**E**) persistent NVD and new preretinal hemorrhage. In general, supplemental treatment is given to areas of the retina not previously treated; however, retreatment over areas that have been previously treated is allowed. (**F**) His proliferative disease regressed completely—note the tight pattern of PRP outside the temporal arcades—and visual acuity was 20/25.

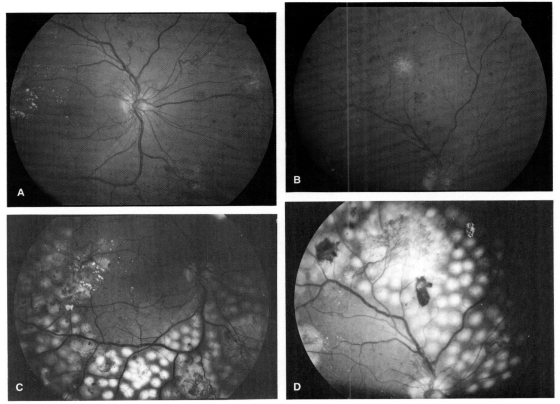

Figure 6–20 A 30-year-old white man, with a 25-year history of insulin-dependent diabetes presented with severe proliferative diabetic retinopathy with (**A**) NVD and (**B**) NVE. The eye received panretinal photocoagulation to the inferior one-half of the retina, with direct treatment of the surface NVE. Although this patient did not have clinically significant macular edema, (**C**) areas of retinal thickening temporal to the foveal avascular zone were also treated with a light grid pattern in conjunction with his panretinal treatment. This was followed 3 weeks later by (**D**) completion of the panretinal photocoagulation to the superior one-half of the retina. Note, that in the ablation of the NVE the vessels are not themselves directly treated, but rather, the underlying retina is confluently treated. (**E**) Six months later, he received supplemental panretinal photocoagulation for residual NVD. (**F**) The patient had recurrent episodes of vitreous hemorrhage, for which he received cryotherapy. (**G**) Regression of his neovascularization and resolution of vitreous hemorrhage is shown.

(continued)

Another use of cryotherapy is in conjunction with laser photocoagulation. If the vitreous hemorrhage is dispersed, but still allows some view of the retina, especially superiorly, laser photocoagulation is attempted first to the superior retina and to any other visible areas with krypton red laser. Then, during the same session cryotreatment is applied to the inferior one-half of the retina, which in general is obscured by the vitreous blood when the patient is sitting in the upright position (Fig. 6-24).

Although limbal conjunctival peritomy is de-

scribed,[45,48] we do not generally use this approach for the first cryotherapy session. If repeat or supplemental cryotherapy is required, the open conjunctival approach with a 360° peritomy will enable the cryoprobe to reach farther posteriorly. We usually do not loop the rectus muscles for retinal cryotherapy treatments during the open conjunctival approach.

Patients should be apprised that they will generally have significant pain following 360° peripheral retinal cryotherapy. Narcotic analgesics, such as acetaminophen with codeine,

(continued on page 104)

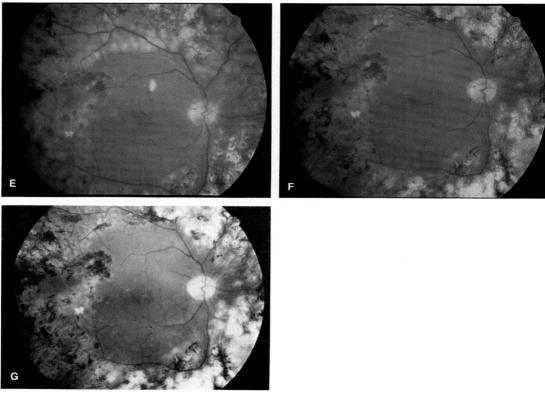

Figure 6–20   (continued)

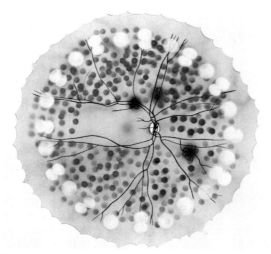

Figure 6–21   Transscleral peripheral cryotherapy. Typical peripheral panretinal cryotherapy is applied with nine lesions in each quadrant for 360°; two lesions are placed at each clock hour, and one lesion is placed at each half-hour from the anterior equator to the ora serrata. In this artist's illlustration, peripheral retinal cryotherapy lesions are placed anterior to the scars of the previous photocoagulation as supplemental treatment.

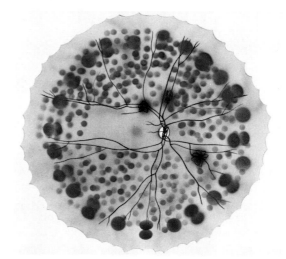

Figure 6–22   Diagrammatic illustration of an eye 2 months after receiving supplemental panretinal photocoagulation and cryotherapy. Note the peripheral confluence of the retinal burns. This patient may complain of peripheral visual field constriction.

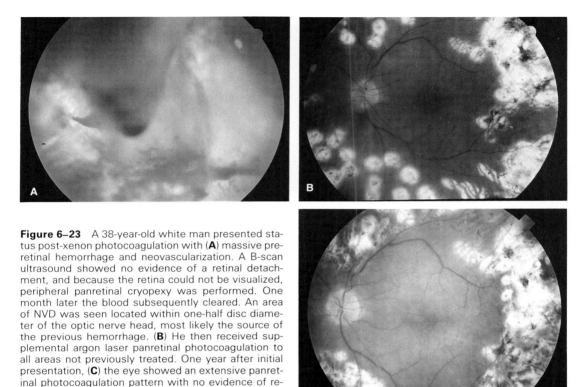

Figure 6–23   A 38-year-old white man presented status post-xenon photocoagulation with (**A**) massive preretinal hemorrhage and neovascularization. A B-scan ultrasound showed no evidence of a retinal detachment, and because the retina could not be visualized, peripheral panretinal cryopexy was performed. One month later the blood subsequently cleared. An area of NVD was seen located within one-half disc diameter of the optic nerve head, most likely the source of the previous hemorrhage. (**B**) He then received supplemental argon laser panretinal photocoagulation to all areas not previously treated. One year after initial presentation, (**C**) the eye showed an extensive panretinal photocoagulation pattern with no evidence of residual neovascularization.

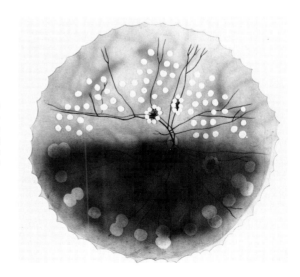

Figure 6–24   Laser photocoagulation with cryotherapy for preretinal or vitreous hemorrhage. First, laser photocoagulation is applied to all areas of visible retina with the krypton red wavelength, mainly superiorly. At the same session, the patient then receives cryotherapy to the inferior one-half of the retina, which is obscured by the vitreous hemorrhage.

or even overnight hospitalization may be required for adequate pain control.

RUBEOSIS AND NEOVASCULAR GLAUCOMA

The efficacy of panretinal photocoagulation in the management of neovascular glaucoma has been demonstrated by several studies.[44,46,48] Early treatment of rubeosis before the development of rubeotic glaucoma yields the most favorable prognosis, and panretinal photocoagulation and cryotherapy, if needed, should be initiated urgently.[15,44,46,48] The iris and angle should be examined under magnification, and the angle configuration should be studied with careful attention to the amount of angle closure. Also, the visual potential must be assessed; an eye with no light perception vision is treated in a manner different from an eye with the potential of even 20/200 vision.

In the early stages of rubeosis following complete panretinal photocoagulation, total regression of the rubeotic vessels may occur and intraocular pressure may remain normal. If the angle is predominantly open in early rubeotic glaucoma following effective photocoagulation and cryotreatment, the glaucoma may be managed medically. Direct photocoagulation of the angle vessels crossing the trabecular meshwork may also be effective. If more than 270° of the angle is closed, however, and if there is potential for useful vision, more than the retinal ablation by panretinal photocoagulation and cryotherapy is needed.

We currently work with the glaucoma service and recommend filtration surgery, often using filtration implants, such as a Molteno implant. Another alternative is cyclodestructive treatment, but if possible, we prefer to save the outflow and filtration apparatus as much as possible. If there is either no vision or bare light perception vision, cyclodestructive procedures are employed to alleviate the patients' discomfort, and patients are then managed medically for palliative measures. It is still important to maximize the visual potential, especially since diabetic patients often have concurrent rubeotic disease in the fellow eye, and

it may be difficult to tell which eye will eventually be the better or worse eye. Once rubeosis is noted, and any visual potential is noted, panretinal photocoagulation or cryotherapy should be promptly instituted in an effort to theoretically control the elaboration of the angiogenic factors responsible for the anterior neovascularization.

EARLY PROLIFERATIVE RETINOPATHY

Clear-cut indications for the treatment of high-risk retinopathy have been defined by the DRS. The management of early proliferative disease is not as unequivocally described. At the 1991 meeting of the American Academy of Ophthalmology and in the 1991 ETDRS reports,[49–51] patients with early proliferative and severe nonproliferative (less than high-risk) retinopathy could be considered for early photocoagulation. Early treatment of these non–high-risk eyes had a small reduction in their rate of severe visual loss (2.6%) compared with controls (3.7%) at 5 years' follow-up. Furthermore, the risk of vitrectomy and progression of retinopathy was reduced by early treatment. However, the side effects of reduced peripheral visual field and early moderate visual loss, most likely caused by exacerbation of preexisting macular edema by scatter photocoagulation, need to be considered in treating eyes with early proliferative disease; this consideration in the decision-making process is made here, since the rates of severe visual loss in this group were so low.

When grading retinopathy in those eyes assigned to the deferral of treatment, looking specifically at their rate of progression to high-risk retinopathy, 21% of eyes with early proliferative disease at 1 year, 49% of eyes at 3 years, and 63% of eyes at 5 years had developed high-risk retinopathy.[50,51] When one considers that, in the DRS, up to 20% of eyes treated at this high-risk stage had severe visual loss, despite adequate photocoagulation,[8] earlier intervention with its attendant lower rate of severe visual loss, as documented in the ETDRS, may be warranted[49,50] (Figs. 6-25 and 6-26).

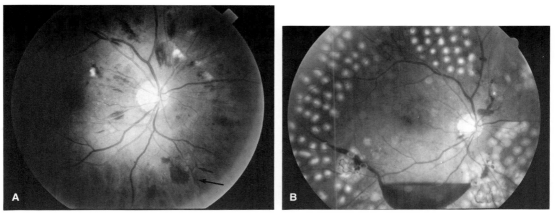

Figure 6–25 This patient presented with (**A**) early proliferative diabetic retinopathy with NVE (*arrow*), cotton-wool spots, and retinal hemorrhages in four quadrants. There was no evidence of NVD. The patient returned 2 months later with (**B**) increased NVE and a boat-shaped preretinal hemorrhage inferiorly and panretinal photocoagulation was performed. Areas of NVE inferior to optic nerve and inferotemporally were treated with confluent ablation. Note that the laser burns are brought no closer than two disc diameters to the temporal edge of the fovea and that direct treatment of the preretinal hemorrhage is avoided. The patient returned 3 weeks later for completion of his panretinal photocoagulation peripheral to the original central zone (not shown).

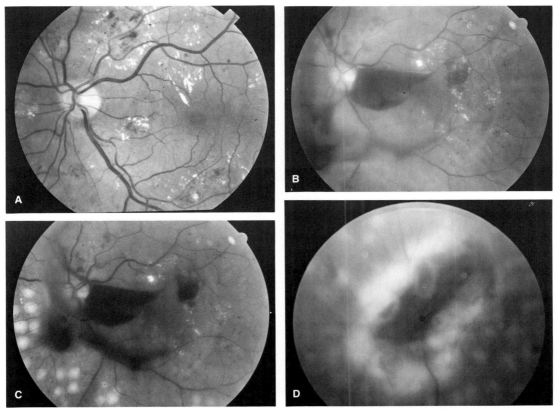

Figure 6–26 A 38-year-old white man who presented with (**A**) severe nonproliferative disease and visual acuity of 20/30. Note the venous beading and IRMA, especially inferotemporally. Four years later, he returned with decreased visual acuity of 20/50 and proliferative diabetic retinopathy. (**B**) Fundus examination showed evidence of new vessels, with subhyaloid and vitreous hemorrhage. (**C**) The patient was treated with krypton red photocoagulation during his first session of panretinal photocoagulation to the inferior half of the retina. (**D**) Panretinal photocoagulation to the superior half of the retina, with confluent ablation to areas of NVE, was completed 3 weeks later, allowing some resorption of the hemorrhage.

105

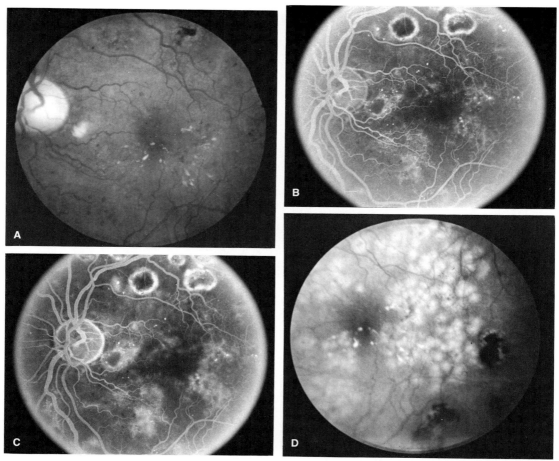

Figure 6–27 This patient presented with diabetic macular edema status postpanretinal xenon laser photocoagulation for proliferative diabetic retinopathy 5 years previously. (**A–C**) Fluorescein angiography showed an irregular and slightly enlarged avascular zone, with diffuse leakage. (**D**) She received modified grid laser treatment to areas of retinal thickening temporal to the fovea as well as superonasal and inferonasal to the foveal avascular zone. (**E,F**) Three months later there was persistent central thickening. (**G**) The patient received supplemental modified grid treatment, and the macular edema resolved. One year later, (**H**) new NVD was noted greater than standard 10A. In addition, central macular edema had recurred and, therefore, the patient underwent (**I**) combined treatment with supplemental grid and (**J**) supplemental panretinal photocoagulation to the inferior one-half of the retina. (**K**) This was followed two weeks later by panretinal photocoagulation to the superior one-half. (**L**) Three months after the supplemental panretinal photocoagulation treatment, there was persistent NVD that had not changed from her preoperative state, and (**M**) the patient underwent an additional session of supplemental panretinal photocoagulation of 1000 burns.

(continued)

A prudent approach then would be to compare the amount of retinopathy in each eye. If one eye has early proliferative disease and the fellow eye has only minimal-to-mild nonproliferative disease, postponing treatment of the early proliferative disease would be appropriate. If the fellow eye has equal retinopathy or worse, early treatment of one eye and then following its response and course can help determine the management of that fellow eye. Once high-risk retinopathy is seen, prompt photocoagulation should be instituted. Thus, the treatment of early proliferative disease is not as clear-cut as that of high-risk retinopathy, but, again, requires an individualized approach (Figs. 6-27 through 6-29).

(continued on page 113)

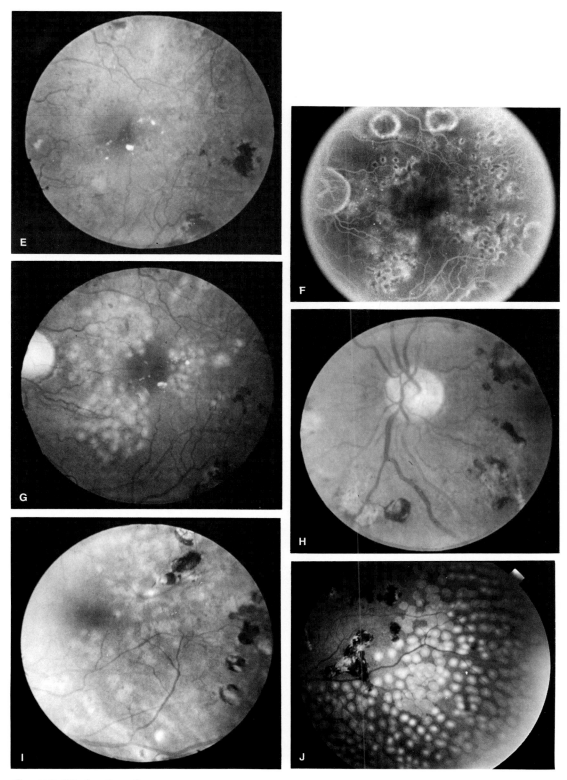

Figure 6–27 (continued)

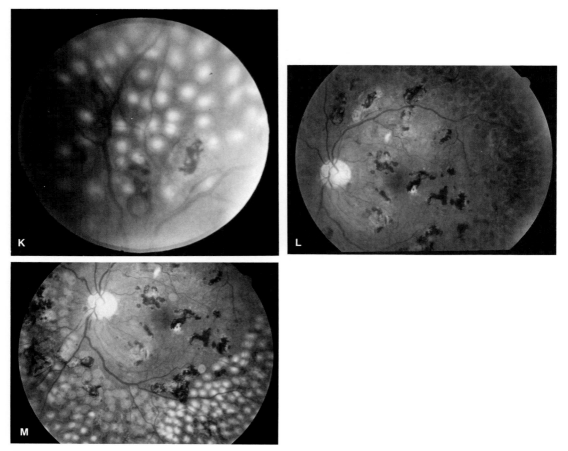

Figure 6–27   (continued)

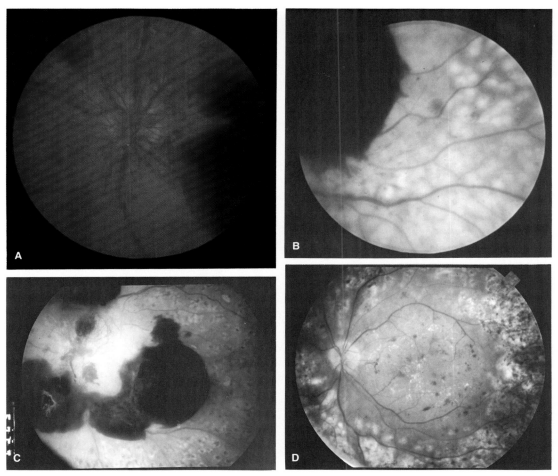

Figure 6-28 A 34-year-old type I insulin-dependent diabetic of 17 years duration, status post below-the-knee amputation, presented with (**A**) severe high-risk retinopathy with massive NVD and preretinal hemorrhage. Visual acuity was 20/800 in the left eye. (**B**) He underwent panretinal photocoagulation to the inferior one-half of the retina, followed 1 month later by the superior one-half. (**C**) The vitreous and subhyaloid hemorrhages had cleared somewhat, but given the extensive NVD, supplemental panretinal photocoagulation was added. He ultimately underwent vitrectomy, combined with membrane delamination and endophotocoagulation, and (**D-F**) over the next 6 months, his proliferative disease involuted, but he developed diffuse diabetic macular edema. (**G**) He underwent modified grid macular treatment. (**H**) Six months later, his diabetic macular edema had resolved, and the central retina was flat. (**I**) Two years later, he had complete regression of his proliferative disease and maculopathy. Visual acuity was 20/200. Six months later, the patient died at age 38 of complications owing to diabetes and hypertension out of control.

(continued)

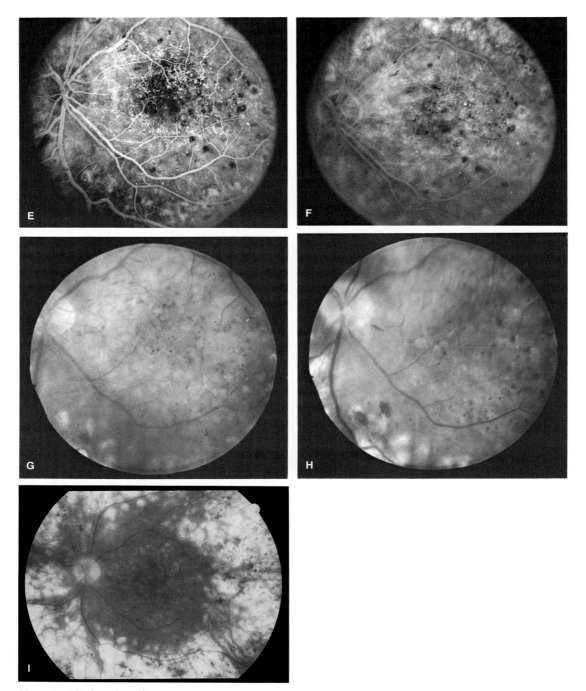

Figure 6–28   (continued)

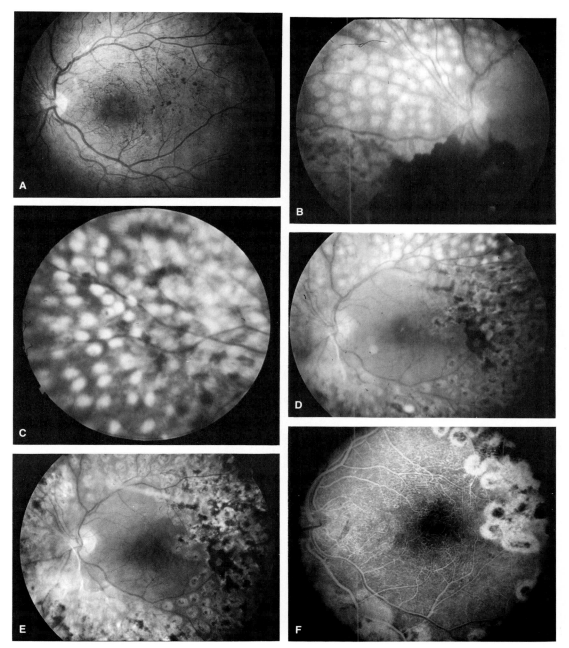

Figure 6–29 A 16-year-old girl presented with (**A**) high-risk proliferative diabetic retinopathy. She was treated with two sessions of panretinal photocoagulation. In between sessions, she developed (**B**) a large vitreous hemorrhage inferiorly, which, however, allowed visualization of the superior retina and completion of the panretinal photocoagulation. Four months later she had a recurrent vitreous hemorrhage, and (**C,D**) supplemental panretinal photocoagulation was added in two sessions to all areas not previously treated. (**E–G**) Six months later her proliferative disease had stabilized, but she developed diffuse diabetic macular edema with cystoid changes. (**H**) She received modified grid photocoagulation. (**I–K**) Four months later her macular edema had resolved, and (**L**) 2 years after initial presentation she has no evidence of recurrent proliferative disease or macular edema. Visual acuity is 20/20.

(continued)

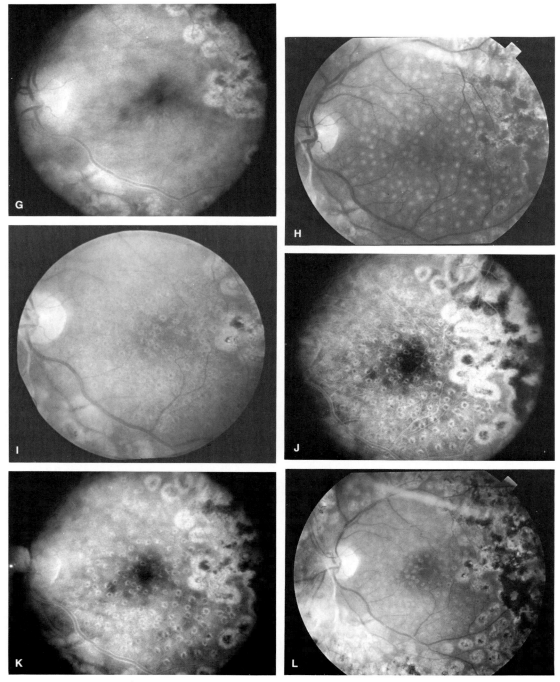

Figure 6–29 (continued)

References

1. National Society to Prevent Blindness, Operational Research Department. Vision problems in the US: A statistical analysis. New York: National Society to Prevent Blindness; 1980: 1–46.
2. Klein R, Klein BEK, Moss SE, Davis MD, DeMets DL. The Wisconsin Epidemiologic Study of Diabetic Retinopathy. II. Prevalence and risk of diabetic retinopathy when age at diagnosis is less than 30 years. Arch Ophthalmol 1984; 102:520–526.
3. Klein R, Klein BEK, Moss SE, Davis MD, DeMets DL. The Wisconsin Epidemiologic Study of Diabetic Retinopathy. III. Prevalence and risk of diabetic retinopathy when age at diagnosis is 30 or more years. Arch Ophthalmol 1984; 102:527–532.
4. Witkin SR, Klein R. Ophthalmologic care for persons with diabetes. JAMA 1984; 251:2534–2537.
5. Klein R, Klein BEK, Moss SE, Davis MD, DeMets DL. The Wisconsin Epidemiologic Study of Diabetic Retinopathy. VI. Retinal photocoagulation. Ophthalmology 1987; 94:747–753.
6. Klein R, Klein BEK, Moss SE, Davis MD, DeMets DL. The Wisconsin Epidemiologic Study of Diabetic Retinopathy. VIII. The incidence of retinal photocoagulation. J Diabetic Complications 1988; 2:79–87.
7. Diabetic Retinopathy Study Research Group. Preliminary report on effects of photocoagulation therapy. Am J Ophthalmol 1976; 81:383–396.
8. Diabetic Retinopathy Study Research Group. Photocoagulation treatment of proliferative diabetic retinopathy: the second report of diabetic retinopathy/vitrectomy study findings. Am J Ophthalmol 1978; 85:82–106.
9. Diabetic Retinopathy Study Research Group. Report no 3. Four risk factors for severe visual loss in diabetic retinopathy. Arch Ophthalmol 1979; 97:654–655.
10. Diabetic Retinopathy Study Research Group. Report no 7. A modification of the Airlie House classification of diabetic retinopathy. Invest Ophthalmol Vis Sci 1981; 21 (part 2):21:210–226.
11. Diabetic Retinopathy Study Research Group. Report no 14. Indications for photocoagulation treatment of diabetic retinopathy. Int Ophthalmol Clin 1987; 27: 239–252.
12. American Academy of Ophthalmology. Preferred practice pattern. Diabetic retinopathy. San Francisco: The American Academy of Ophthalmology 1989.
13. Jacobson DR, Murphy RD, Rosenthal AR. The treatment of angle neovascularization with panretinal photocoagulation. Ophthalmology 1979; 86:1270–1277.
14. Pavan PR, Folk JC. Anterior neovascularization. Int Ophthalmol Clin 1984; 24:61–70.
15. Murphy RP, Egbert PR. Regression of iris neovascularization following panretinal photocoagulation. Arch Ophthalmol 1979; 97:700.
16. Plumb AP, Swan AV, Chignell AH, Shilling JS. A comparative trial of xenon arc and argon laser photocoagulation in the treatment of proliferative diabetic retinopathy. Br J Ophthalmol 1982; 66:213–218.
17. Hamilton AM, Townsend C, Khoury D, et al. Xenon arc and argon laser photocoagulation in the treatment of diabetic disc neovascularization. Part 1: effect on disc vessels, visual fields, and visual acuity. Trans Ophthalmol Soc UK 1981; 101:87–92.
18. Mainster MA. Wavelength selection in macular photocoagulation: tissue optics, thermal effects, and laser systems. Ophthalmology 1986; 93:952–958.
19. Early Treatment Diabetic Retinopathy Study Research Group. Report no 3. Techniques for scatter and local photocoagulation treatment of diabetic retinopathy. Int Ophthalmol Clin 1987; 27:254–264.
20. Olk RJ. Argon green (514 nm) versus krypton red (647 nm) modified grid laser photocoagulation for diffuse diabetic macular edema. Ophthalmology 1990; 97:1101–1113.
21. Crues AF, Williams JC, Willan AR. Argon green and krypton red laser treatment of diabetic macular edema. Can J Ophthalmol 1988; 23:262–266.
22. Casswell AG, Canning CR, Gregor ZJ. Treatment of diffuse diabetic macular edema: a comparison between argon and krypton lasers. Eye 1990; 4:668–672.
23. Schulenberg WE, Hamilton AM, Blach RK. A comparative study of argon laser and krypton lasers in the treatment of diabetic optic disc neovascularization. Br J Ophthalmol 1979; 63:412–417.
24. Blankenship GW. Red krypton and blue-green argon panretinal laser photocoagulation for proliferative diabetic retinopathy: a laboratory and clinical comparison. Am Ophthalmol Soc 1986; 84:967–1003.
25. Singerman LJ, et al. Krypton laser for proliferative diabetic retinopathy: the krypton argon regression of neovascularization study. J Diabetic Complications 1988; 2:189–196.
26. The Krypton-Argon Regression Neovascularization Study Research Group. Randomized comparison of krypton versus argon scatter photocoagulation for diabetic disc neovascularization. Ophthalmology 1993; 100:1655–1664.
27. Reddy VM, Zamora R, Olk RJ. A comparison of the size of the burn produced by Rodenstock and Goldmann contact lenses. Am J Ophthalmol 1991; 112:212–214.
28. Barr CC. Estimation of the maximum number of argon laser burns possible in panretinal photocoagulation. Am J Ophthalmol 1984; 97:697–703.
29. Doft BH, Blankenship GW. Single versus multiple treatment sessions of argon laser panretinal photocoagulation for proliferative diabetic retinopathy. Ophthalmology 1982; 89:772–779.
30. Rogell GD. Incremental panretinal photocoagulation. Retina 1984; 3:308–311.
31. Doft BH, Blankenship G. Retinopathy risk factor regression after laser panretinal photocoagulation for proliferative diabetic retinopathy. Ophthalmology 1984; 91:1453–1457.
32. Blankenship GW. A clinical comparison of central and peripheral argon laser panretinal photocoagu-

lation for proliferative diabetic retinopathy. Ophthalmology 1988; 95:170–177.

33. McDonald HR, Schatz H. Visual loss following panretinal photocoagulation for proliferative diabetic retinopathy. Ophthalmology 1985; 92:388–393.

34. Shimizu K, Kobayaski Y, Muraoka K. Midperipheral fundus involvement in diabetic retinopathy. Ophthalmology 1981; 88:601–612.

35. Niki T, Muraoka K, Shimizu K. Distribution of capillary nonperfusion in early-stage diabetic retinopathy. Ophthalmology 1984; 91:1431–1439.

36. Patz A. Clinical and experimental studies on retinal neovascularization, 39th Edward Jackson Memorial Lecture. Am J Ophthalmol 1982; 94:715–743.

37. Bresnick GH. Background diabetic retinopathy. In: Ryan S, ed. Retina, vol 2. St. Louis: CV Mosby Co, 1989:327–366.

38. Diabetic Retinopathy Study Research Group. Report no 8. Photocoagulation of proliferative diabetic retinopathy: clinical applications of DRS findings. Invest Ophthalmol Vis Sci 1981; 88:583–600.

39. Vine AK. The efficacy of additional argon laser photocoagulation for persistent, severe proliferative diabetic retinopathy. Ophthalmology 1985; 92:1532–1537.

40. Boniuk I, Johnston GP, Arribas NP, Escoffery RF. Supplementary peripheral photocoagulation in the treatment of proliferative diabetic retinopathy. Mod Probl Ophthalmol 1979; 20:401–406.

41. Vander JF, Duker JS, Benson WE, et al. Long-term stability and visual outcome after favorable initial response of proliferative diabetic retinopathy to panretinal photocoagulation. Ophthalmology 1991; 98:1575–1579.

42. Ramsay WJ, Ramsay RC, Purple RL, Knobloch WH.

Involutional diabetic retinopathy. Am J Ophthalmol 1977; 84:851–858.

43. Schimek RA, Spencer R. Cryopexy treatment of proliferative diabetic retinopathy: retinal cryoablation in patients with severe vitreous hemorrhage. Arch Ophthalmol 1979; 97:1276–1280.

44. Hilton GF. Panretinal cryotherapy for diabetic rubeosis [Letter]. Arch Ophthalmol 1979; 97:776.

45. Daily MJ, Geiser RG. Treatment of proliferative diabetic retinopathy with panretinal cryotherapy. Ophthalmol Surg 1984; 15:741–745.

46. Brodell LP, Olk RJ, Arribas NP, et al. Neovascular glaucoma: a retrospective analysis of treatment with peripheral panretinal cryotherapy. Ophthalmol Surg 1987; 18:200–206.

47. Benedett R, Olk RJ, Arribas NP, et al. Transconjunctival anterior retinal cryotherapy for proliferative diabetic retinopathy. Ophthalmology 1987; 94:612–619.

48. May DR, Bergstrom TJ, Parmet AJ, Schwartz JG. Treatment of neovascular glaucoma with transscleral panretinal cryotherapy. Ophthalmology 1980; 87:1106–1111.

49. Early Treatment Diabetic Retinopathy Study Research Group. Report no 7. Early treatment diabetic retinopathy study design and baseline patient characteristics. Ophthalmology 1991; 98:741–756.

50. Early Treatment Diabetic Retinopathy Research Group. Report no 9. Early photocoagulation for diabetic retinopathy. Ophthalmology 1991; 98:766–785.

51. Early Treatment Diabetic Retinopathy Research Group. Report no 12. Fundus photographic risk factors for progression of diabetic retinopathy. Ophthalmology 1991; 98:823–833.

Diabetic Retinopathy: Practical Management, by R. Joseph Olk and Carol M. Lee. J.B. Lippincott Company, Philadelphia © 1993.

C H A P T E R · 7

Indications for Vitrectomy

The indications for vitrectomy in the management of diabetic retinopathy have evolved since 1970, when Machemer first introduced this modality for the treatment of diabetic vitreous hemorrhage.[1] The removal of the vitreous blood provided, in many instances, the restoration of some vision and, at the same time, removed the framework upon which fibrovascular proliferation occurred.

The natural course of neovascular tissue has been shown to reflect its intimate arrangement and dependence on the vitreous framework. Clinical observation shows that patches of new vessels are relatively flat or minimally raised before posterior vitreous detachment and that the new vessels appear to be adherent to the posterior vitreous surface. As the posterior hyaloid detaches, it pulls up the adherent new vessels, elevating and breaking the new vessels, causing hemorrhage. The posterior hyaloid can continue to detach, but points of adherence between the vitreous and neovascular stalks are often seen precluding complete posterior vitreous detachment. The posterior hyaloid face that has detached undergoes contraction and, with the fibrovascular component still growing along the surface from the points of attachment, will cause traction of the underlying retinal tissue.[2,3] This epiretinal traction and the anteroposterior traction between the posterior hyaloid and the new vessels growing from the disc and retinal surface must be eliminated to relieve the retinal tissues from tractional elevation. Thus, not only must the blood be removed, but the tractional forces also need to be severed to restore the anatomy and function of the retina.

VITREOUS HEMORRHAGE

Vitrectomy for vitreous hemorrhage is a well-studied indication[1,4–8] and was, in the early days of vitreous surgery, the most common indication for vitrectomy in diabetes.[1,8] As discussed in Chapter 3, the Diabetic Retinopathy Vitrectomy Study (DRVS) reported on the 2- and 4-year follow-up results for patients undergoing vitrectomy for vitreous hemorrhage from the standpoint of the timing of surgery relative to outcome.[9–13] Group H consisted of eyes with severe vitreous hemorrhage of less than 5 months' duration and visual acuity of ≤ 5/200 with enough blood to obscure fundus details on clinical examination. These group H eyes were randomized to *early vitrectomy,* defined in the study as 1 month from randomization, or deferred until 1 year after the onset of hemorrhage. Surgery was performed on deferral eyes before the 1-year interval if tractional detachment of the macula occurred, and it was performed after 1 year for either macular detachment or persistent nonclearing hemorrhage.

The DRVS found that early vitrectomy for severe vitreous hemorrhage was significantly associated with attainment of better vision and better anatomic results at both the 2- and 4-year follow-up visits in eyes of younger patients with type I diabetes, defined here as age at diagnosis of insulin-requiring diabetes of no older than 20 years.[10,13] No significant difference in visual or anatomic outcome was attributed to timing of vitrectomy in either type II patients (defined as patients whose age of diagnosis of diabetes is 40 years or older or whose diabetes is non–insulin-requiring) or in the mixed group patients (defined as patients whose age of diagnosis of insulin-requiring diabetes was between 21 and 39 years).

TRACTIONAL RETINAL DETACHMENT

Diabetic tractional retinal detachment involving the macula is currently the most common cause of vitrectomy for diabetic disease.[8,14] It replaced vitreous hemorrhage as the most frequent cause for surgery, most likely because of the extensive use of panretinal photocoagulation. As the fibrovascular tissue within the neo-

vascular complex continues to contract, concurrent with a partial posterior hyaloidal detachment, the connections within this complex to the retina cause progressive tractional detachment of the retina itself. Often the posterior vitreous detachment occurs after the fibrovascular tissue has grown along the posterior vitreous surface. As the detachment of the vitreous progresses, the retina is slowly elevated by connections most often along the arcades and the optic disc. However, extramacular traction detachments can be quite stable; the incidence of progression to involve the macula is only about 14% at 1 year, 21% at 2 years, and 23% at 3 years.[15,16] Patients who have extramacular traction detachments are followed closely at about 3-month intervals if they are symptomatically stable. Patients are advised to return immediately for repeat evaluation if any loss of vision is noted (Figs. 7-1 and 7-2).

Surgery is not routinely indicated for an extramacular traction detachment, but once the macula is affected, prompt intervention is recommended. Delaying surgery for a long period may allow irreversible changes to occur within the macular retinal tissues (Figs. 7-3 and 7-4). When traction ·detachment of the macula occurs, significant epiretinal membranes are usually present. With modern bimanual vitreoretinal techniques, the membrane can be approached in one of several ways: Following complete removal of the vitreous and posterior hyaloid, the fibrovascular bundles and residual

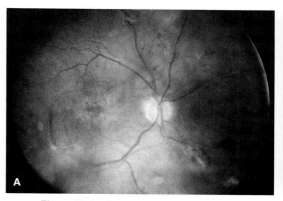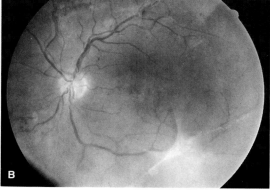

Figure 7–1   An example of bilateral extramacular traction retinal detachment is shown. Vitrectomy surgery here is not indicated, and close follow-up is recommended for this patient.

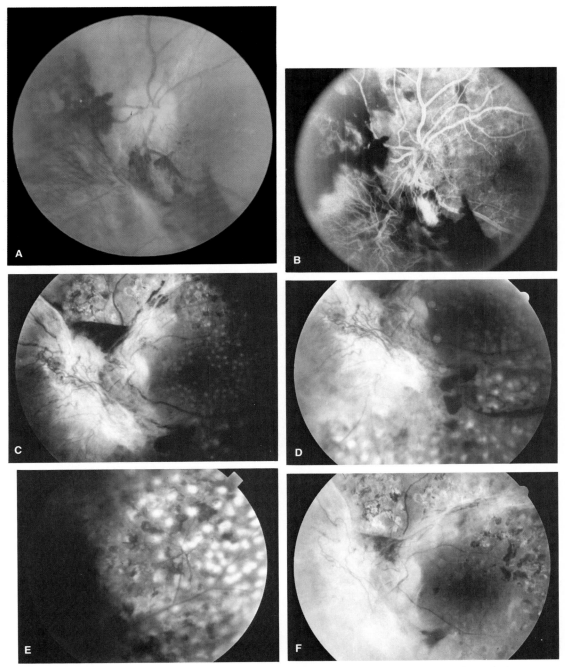

Figure 7–2 A 42-year-old black woman, status post-panretinal photocoagulation performed elsewhere 2 years before presentation and with 16-years duration of type II diabetes, presented with (**A**) traction detachment inferiorly, preretinal hemorrhage, and (**B**) severe proliferative disease and extensive capillary nonperfusion, with macular edema. The macular area itself was not threatened by the traction retinal detachment, and (**C,D**) supplemental panretinal photocoagulation combined with modified grid photocoagulation to the macula was recommended. Note that the photocoagulation spots were placed to avoid direct treatment over the areas of fibrosis, and all areas of previously untreated retina are now treated. (**E**) She received more supplemental panretinal photocoagulation, and 4 months later no new hemorrhage was present; (**F**) the traction detachment remained stable, and the macular edema had resolved. As her macula was not threatened by the traction retinal detachment, laser photocoagulation was used as an initial treatment option, rather than vitrectomy surgery.

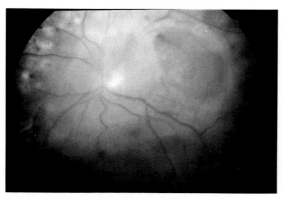

Figure 7–3   A macular traction retinal detachment. The patient is status post-panretinal photocoagulation for proliferative diabetic retinopathy. Vitrectomy and delamination of the posterior hyaloid were recommended for this patient.

vitreoretinal adhesions are lysed to relieve the tangential retinal-to-retinal traction. Usually vertically oriented scissors are employed to segment the fibrovascular membranes between epicenters, and horizontally oriented scissors are employed to delaminate the residual membrane from the surface of the epicenters and underlying blood vessels.[1,14,17–20] Segmentation can leave residual islands of fibrovascular tissue, which could possibly reproliferate and cause new tangential epiretinal traction, rebleed, or obscure underlying retinal lesions (Fig. 7-5).

Another method of completely removing the fibrovascular membranes involves the "en bloc

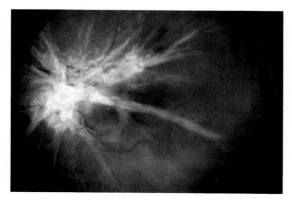

Figure 7–4   This is a 37-year-old black man with a 20-year history of insulin-dependent diabetes. This is an example of a macular traction retinal detachment and extensive fibrosis over the optic nerve.

method,"[21,22] which uses the anteroposterior traction of the posterior hyaloid attachment to the retina to aid in the removal of the fibrovascular complex, with the posterior hyaloid, as a single entity. Here, horizontally oriented scissors are used to separate the hyaloid and contiguous fibrovascular membranes from the retina through an opening made in the posterior hyaloid. After separating the retinal attachments to the fibrovascular complex, using the attached posterior hyaloid for additional stabilization, the membranes are lifted from the retinal surface, and the entire hyaloidal–fibrovascular membranes, which have been freed, are excised as a unit with the vitrectomy instrument. The methods chosen are determined by the anatomic surgical presentation; any and all of these methods described may be employed during a single procedure. Further discussion of the surgical technique is beyond the scope of this chapter, and the reader is advised to consult any of several textbooks on vitrectomy surgery (Fig. 7-6).

TRACTIONAL–RHEGMATOGENOUS RETINAL DETACHMENT

Another indication for surgical intervention is the presence of a combined traction–rhegmatogenous retinal detachment.[22–24] Full-thickness retinal defects can develop because the retina is subject to traction from the vitreoretinal adhesions in both an anteroposterior direction from the retina to the vitreous base and tangentially between the epicenters of fibrovascular proliferation parallel to the surface of the retina. Vitrectomy and membrane dissection permit identification of the retinal breaks; all surrounding retinal traction must be alleviated. Air–fluid exchange can then be performed through the retinal hole or holes and sealed with either endophotocoagulation, diathermy, or cryotreatment. Intraocular gas is then used to tamponade the retina until chorioretinal adhesion takes place. In general, if the retinal breaks can be approached with internal tamponade, we prefer to manage these

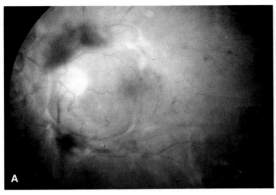 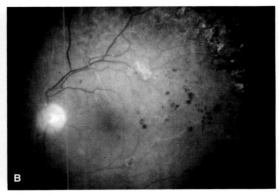

Figure 7–5 A 42-year-old status post-panretinal photocoagulation patient presented with sudden loss of vision, visual acuity of 20/400, and (**A**) a macular traction retinal detachment involving the inferotemporal and superotemporal arcades. (**B**) She underwent vitrectomy, with membrane delamination and segmentation, and 3 months postoperatively her visual acuity had returned to 20/40. Note the complete flattening of the macula and posterior pole and two small residual islands of fibrous tissue along both the superotemporal and inferotemporal arcades.

breaks internally. If the breaks are located peripherally, lending themselves to repair with an external scleral buckle, this method is then used to push the retinal hole against the retinal pigment epithelium.

Prophylactic scleral buckles are no longer routinely used in the management of tractional detachments and are only occasionally used in the management of combination rhegmatogenous and tractional diabetic detachments, since it has been our experience and that of other authors[25,26] that the placement of prophylactic scleral buckles has been significantly associated with the development of anterior hyaloidal proliferation following diabetic vitrectomy. Although we cannot determine whether the scleral buckle itself directly causes anterior hyaloidal disease, anterior retinal perfusion may be compromised by compression on the vortex venous and choroidal systems,[27] further compromising the already ischemic retinal tissue.[25–27]

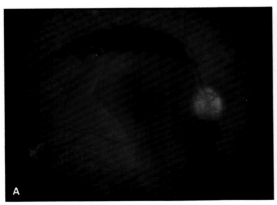 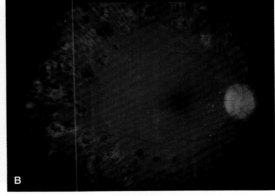

Figure 7–6 A 35-year-old insulin-dependent diabetic, status post-multiple sessions of panretinal photocoagulation and cryotherapy (**A**) now presents with recurrent NVD, vitreous hemorrhage, and subhyaloid hemorrhage over the posterior pole. Visual acuity is count-fingers. No clearing was noted over 6 weeks. She underwent trans-pars plana vitrectomy, with membrane delamination, removal of the subhyaloid blood, and endolaser photocoagulation. One year after surgery, visual acuity was 20/40, without (**B**) evidence of any proliferative disease.

SEVERE PROLIFERATIVE DIABETIC RETINOPATHY

As indicated in the beginning of this chapter, advances made in modern vitreoretinal techniques in the last two decades have allowed successful surgical intervention for a variety of reasons other than those previously discussed. Severe proliferative retinopathy, despite good vision, is an indication for surgical intervention.[8,28] The DRVS[11,12] looked at eyes with extensive active neovascular or fibrovascular proliferations, with best corrected visual acuity of 10/200 or better, which were randomized to either early vitrectomy or conventional management with serial clinical follow-up. They found that at both the 2- and 4-year follow-up visits, eyes that were randomized to early vitrectomy had an increased and sustained chance of achieving 10/20 vision or better; eyes with more severe proliferative disease showed the greatest beneficial treatment effect. Other studies[28] have also shown that early vitrectomy is efficacious in maintaining vision and preventing further visual loss in eyes with severe fibrovascular proliferation. We recommend that maximal panretinal photocoagulation be first applied to selected patients in whom the retina is seen with very severe neovascular and fibrovascular disease. If no significant regression or if rapid progressive traction is seen and, especially, if preretinal or vitreous hemorrhage coexists, early vitrectomy with removal of the fibrovascular membranes should be performed.

OTHER INDICATIONS FOR VITRECTOMY

Another indication for surgical intervention is the coexistence of significant, dense, preretinal hemorrhage, especially overlying the posterior pole.[6,8,29] Although most eyes with preretinal hemorrhage will clear the blood spontaneously and can be managed with extensive panretinal photocoagulation, some eyes with thick preretinal hemorrhage in tight apposition to the macula will develop macular traction. The hemorrhage into the subhyaloid space can cause fibrovascular proliferation and subsequent traction on the macular surface. Progressive traction can lead to macular detachment in this subset of patients. Additionally, prolonged subhyaloid or preretinal hemorrhage within the macular region may potentially cause retinal pigment epithelial and photoreceptor damage.

Thick premacular fibrosis can be seen following extensive panretinal photocoagulation, or subhyaloid hemorrhage overlying the macula.[6,29] If the fibrosis appears to be the cause of visual loss after evaluation, by fluorescein angiography, of the perfusion state of the macula, vitrectomy and membrane peeling may be recommended. Diaphanous epiretinal membranes or wrinkling of the internal limiting membrane is often clinically seen after extensive laser treatment or after resorbed vitreous hemorrhage. Surgical intervention is recommended only if it is felt that significant visual impairment is caused by these membranes.

Indications for reoperation now include recurrent large vitreous hemorrhage,[30] massive postvitrectomy fibrin response,[5,31,32] and progressive anterior hyaloidal proliferation, either originating from the peripheral retina or from the pars plana and extending anteriorly over the ciliary body surface, iris, and lens.[5,33] This condition is very similar to what is referred to as *anterior proliferative vitreoretinopathy*. In diabetic eyes, this process soon leads to neovascular proliferation along the anterior structures of the eye, with the development of iris neovascularization, neovascular glaucoma, and phthisis. It should be addressed promptly with appropriate preoperative photocoagulation or cryotreatment, or both. In these quite advanced cases, membrane dissection needs to be extensive and complete and often requires lensectomy which, in general, is not advocated for routine surgical management of diabetic retinopathy. These very severely damaged eyes carry a poor prognosis and may require the use of silicone oil as an additional tamponade.

The prognosis for patients undergoing vitrectomy for complications of diabetic retinopathy have been studied by various investigators.[4,5,7,9–13,24,34] Certain preoperative characteristics appear to be prognostic indicators associated with a better visual outcome. In one study by Thompson and colleagues in 1987,[34] these favorable characteristics included age at surgery younger than 40; use of insulin at the time of surgery; better preoperative visual acuity; indication for surgery being vitreous hemorrhage, rather than tractional retinal detachment of the macula, or combined rhegmatogenous and tractional retinal detachment; and the absence of use of intraocular gas during surgery, reflecting the absence of retinal hole formation.

In general, the presence of preoperative rubeosis[5,4,34] and the use of lensectomy during surgery[7,34–36] bears a particularly unfavorable prognosis. It is felt that lens removal is associated with an increased incidence of postoperative iris neovascularization and neovascular glaucoma because the lens may act as a natural barrier to vasoproliferative factors released by an ischemic retina. The removal of the lens may then allow free diffusion of these factors into the anterior chamber.

With current vitreoretinal techniques, the DRVS showed that 25% of patients undergoing early vitrectomy for dense, nonclearing vitreous hemorrhage alone can expect visual acuity of 20/40 or better, and up to 40% of patients can expect visual acuity of 20/100 or better.[13] Up to 60% of eyes can expect visual acuity of at least 20/200 after vitrectomy for vitreous hemorrhage alone.[4,5,13,23,24] From 20% to almost 60% of eyes operated on for tractional macular detachment can expect vision of at least 20/200[17,18] and from 10% to 20% may reach postoperative visual acuity of 20/40 or better.[17,18,37] For eyes with severe proliferative retinopathy, but good preoperative visual acuity, up to 44% can maintain visual acuity of 20/40 or better at 4 years' follow-up.[11] Eyes with combined traction–rhegmatogenous detachment have a worse prognosis, however. Approximately 25% to 35% obtain visual acuity of 20/200 or better postoperatively.[22,24]

RECOMMENDATIONS FOR MANAGEMENT

Considerations of individual presentation must be taken into account when surgery is being contemplated. The status of the fellow eye must be considered, especially if the fellow eye is severely damaged to a point that prompt visual rehabilitation might be afforded by surgery. The amount of preoperative photocoagulation should be maximized before surgery, unless a tractional macular detachment is present, in which event, surgery should be performed promptly. The importance of panretinal photocoagulation is stressed here to both address the neovascular process itself and to decrease the risk of postoperative rubeosis and neovascular glaucoma.[35,38,39] When possible, intraoperative endophotocoagulation is also important to diminish the risk of both anterior segment complications and recurrent retinal neovascularization and recurrent vitreous hemorrhage.[8,40] If an eye already has anterior segment rubeosis and has significant vitreous hemorrhage, precluding transpupillary or indirect laser photocoagulation, cryotherapy should be performed, and early vitrectomy should be considered to allow complete retinal ablation by photocoagulation.

Younger-onset insulin-dependent patients with significant vitreous hemorrhage are recommended for early vitrectomy. In general, a waiting period of approximately 1 to 2 months is recommended to see if any clearing occurs. Older-onset insulin and non–insulin-dependent patients who present with a severe vitreous hemorrhage are followed closely at 1-month intervals to watch for both clearing of the hemorrhage and for the development of tractional macular detachment. Serial clinical examinations and echography should be employed if the blood precludes adequate visualization of the posterior pole. Patients are instructed to elevate the head of their bed and avoid heavy bending, lifting, or straining. If an older-onset insulin-dependent or non–insulin-dependent individual shows no significant clearing of the blood in 6 to 12 months with sustained visual impairment, vitrectomy is recommended. However, if the fellow eye has very advanced disease or if the patient is anatomically or functionally monocular, earlier vitrectomy should be considered to provide for visual rehabilitation, after waiting for a few months to see whether spontaneous clearing occurs.

Eyes with massive preretinal hemorrhage, whether in younger or older insulin-dependent or non–insulin-dependent patients, should be followed closely. If no significant clearing is seen or if a fibrovascular response involving the macula with potential macular traction detachment is noted, early surgical intervention can be recommended (Figs. 7-7 and 7-8). Eyes with severe, active neovascular and fibrovascular disease, despite panretinal photocoagulation, should be considered for surgery. With current techniques, removal of the vitreous framework and fibrovascular complex will permit complete photocoagulation either intraoperatively with the endolaser or by indirect laser, or postoperatively with the slit lamp or indirect laser (Fig. 7-9).

In special cases in which the lens is opacified preoperatively and precludes adequate visualization during surgery and adequate visual rehabilitation postoperatively, posterior chamber lens implantation after completion of pars plana lensectomy and vitrectomy can be per-

formed in a single procedure[41] or following the vitrectomy as a second procedure.[42,43] Also, if a posterior capsulotomy is performed intraoperatively, for instance, in the single-stage procedure, intraoperative endophotocoagulation and postoperative panretinal photocoagulation should be maximized at the time of surgery to decrease the risk of postoperative rubeosis.[8,35,36,38–40]

Although the visual outcome and potential for usable vision is quite promising, the risk of surgery must always be weighed against these advantages. Not only must the medical status and anesthetic risk be evaluated, but the patient must also be apprised of the increased risk of developing severe visual loss up to "no light perception" vision. From 5% up to 17% to 25% of eyes undergoing vitrectomy for vitreous hemorrhage,[4,10,13] up to 11% to 19% of eyes undergoing vitrectomy for tractional macular detachment,[17,18,37] and up to 10% to 23% of eyes undergoing vitrectomy for combined traction–rhegmatogenous detachment may lose all light perception after surgery.[22,24] In the DRVS, there were more eyes having no light perception vision during the first 2 years following early vitrectomy for vitreous hemorrhage than in the deferral eyes, but these differences were not significant at the 24-month visit or later. Vitrectomy surgery can also be attended by compli-

(continued on page 126)

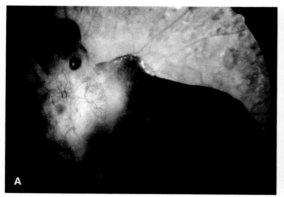 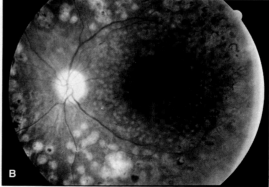

Figure 7–7   A 32-year-old white woman, with insulin-dependent diabetes of 25-years duration, status post-panretinal photocoagulation in the left eye, presented with (**A**) recurrent increasing proliferative diabetic retinopathy and subhyaloid hemorrhage overlying the posterior pole. Visual acuity was count-fingers. The patient underwent vitrectomy and membrane delamination, and over the next 6 years had modified grid and supplemental panretinal photocoagulation. Visual acuity was ultimately 20/20 (**B**) with no evidence of proliferative retinopathy or macular edema.

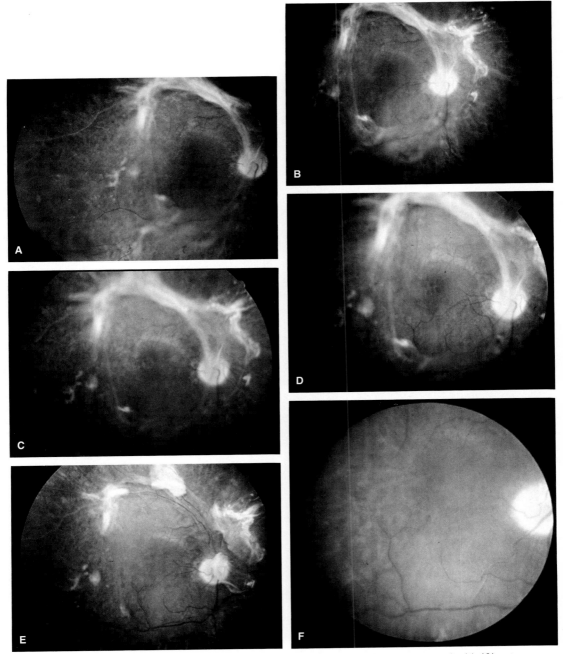

Figure 7–8 A 45-year-old white man, with insulin-dependent diabetes, presented with (**A**) extra-macular traction retinal detachment. (**B**) Over the next year the traction retinal detachment encroached on the macular area. Four months later, (**C**) the patient experienced a spontaneous partial posterior vitreous detachment relieving the tractional component on the macula with improved visual acuity. One year later, increasing fibrosis was noted, causing a recurrent tractional detachment of the posterior pole. (**D**) The macula itself was threatened as the traction extended up to the edge of the fovea, and visual acuity had decreased to 20/400. The patient underwent trans-pars plana vitrectomy and membrane delamination and segmentation. (**E,F**) Note the residual islands of fibrovascular tissue along the superior arcades and that the retina itself is completely flat.

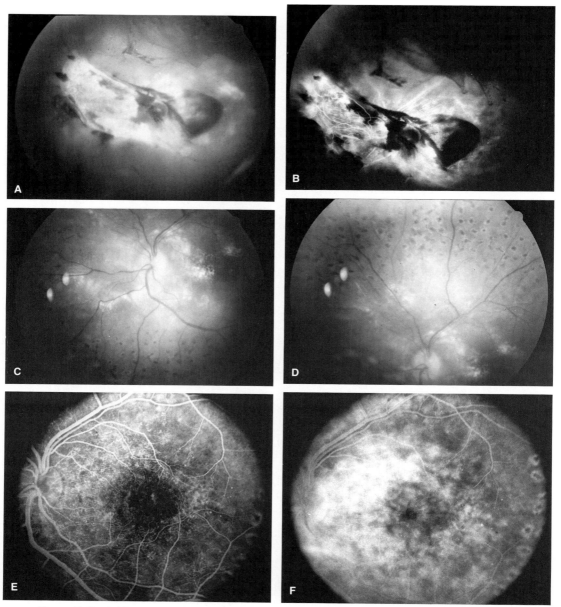

Figure 7–9 A 26-year-old white woman, with type I diabetes of 11-years duration, presented 1 month postpartum with (**A,B**) severe proliferative retinopathy in her left eye with subhyaloid hemorrhage, vitreous hemorrhage, and traction detachment of the posterior pole. Visual acuity was count-fingers at 1.5 m (5 ft). She underwent trans-pars plana vitrectomy, membrane delamination, and endolaser photocoagulation. One month postoperatively there was no evidence of traction detachment of the macula, but macular edema was present, as expected. Visual acuity was 20/200. (**C,D**) Photocoagulation scars are seen in the midperiphery, without evidence of any new bleeding. She was followed over the next several months, and the macular edema persisted. Visual acuity was 20/80. Modified grid photocoagulation was recommended, and (**E,F**) fluorescein angiography was performed. (**G**) Modified grid photocoagulation was applied to areas of retinal thickening. (**H,I**) At 3 months follow-up, she had residual macular edema, as seen on fluorescein angiography, and (**J**) supplemental modified grid treatment was performed. Nine months later, 18 months after the original surgery, her visual acuity was 20/25, and (**K**) she had no evidence of recurrent proliferative disease or residual macular edema.

(continued)

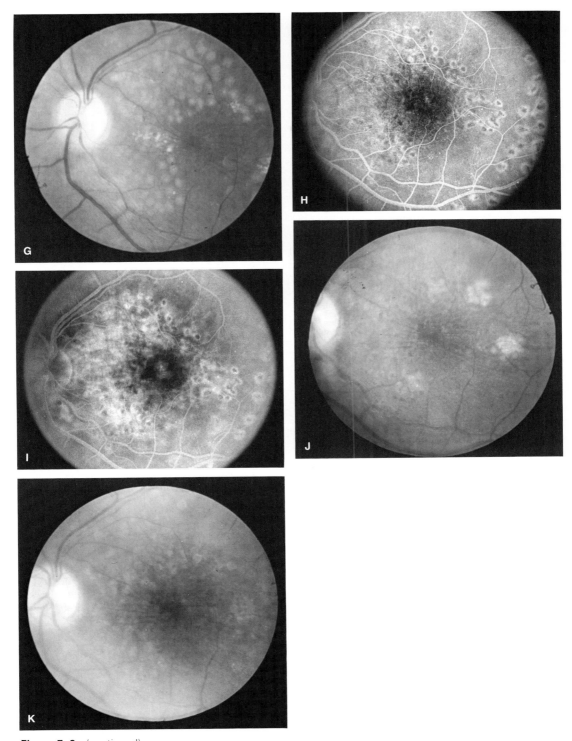

Figure 7–9 (continued)

cations, including endophthalmitis, accelerated cataract formation and, in diabetic patients especially, neovascularization of the iris and neovascular glaucoma. The surgical goals of evacuating the vitreous cavity of blood and removing the anteroposterior traction and epiretinal tangential traction can be achieved with modern techniques, but the decision to recommend vitrectomy in the management of diabetic retinopathy must weigh both the benefits and risks posed to the patient on an individual basis.

References

1. Machemer R, Buettner H, Norton EWD, et al. Vitrectomy: a pars plana approach. Trans Am Acad Ophthalmol Otolaryngol 1971; 75:813–820.
2. Davis MD. Proliferative diabetic retinopathy. In: Ryan SJ, ed. Retina, vol 2. St Louis: CV Mosby Co; 1989: 367–402.
3. Davis MD. Vitreous contraction in proliferative diabetic retinopathy. Arch Ophthalmol 1965; 74:741.
4. Machemer R, Blankenship G. Vitrectomy for proliferative diabetic retinopathy associated with vitreous hemorrhage. Ophthalmology 1981; 88:643–646.
5. Michels RG, Rice TA, Rice EF. Vitrectomy for diabetic vitreous hemorrhage. Am J Ophthalmol 1983; 95: 12–21.
6. Ramsay RC, Knoblock WH, Cantrill HL. Timing of vitrectomy for active proliferative diabetic retinopathy. Ophthalmology 1986; 93:283–289.
7. Blankenship GW, Machemer R. Long-term diabetic vitrectomy results. Report of 10 year follow-up. Ophthalmology 1985; 92:503–506.
8. Aaberg TM, Abrams GW. Changing indications and techniques for vitrectomy in management of complications of diabetic retinopathy. Ophthalmology 1987; 94:775–779.
9. Diabetic Retinopathy Vitrectomy Study Research Group. Report no 1. Two-year course of visual acuity in severe proliferative diabetic retinopathy with conventional management. Ophthalmology 1985; 92:492–502.
10. Diabetic Retinopathy Vitrectomy Study Research Group. Report no 2. Early vitrectomy for severe vitreous hemorrhage in diabetic retinopathy. Two-year results of a randomized trial. Arch Ophthalmol 1985; 103:1644–1652.
11. Diabetic Retinopathy Vitrectomy Study Research Group. Report no 3. Early vitrectomy for severe proliferative diabetic retinopathy in eyes with useful vision. Results of a randomized trial. Ophthalmology 1988; 95:1307–1320.
12. Diabetic Retinopathy Vitrectomy Study Research Group. Report no 4. Early vitrectomy for severe proliferative diabetic retinopathy in eyes with useful vision. Clinical application of results of a randomized trial. Ophthalmology 1988; 95:1321–1334.
13. Diabetic Retinopathy Vitrectomy Study Research Group. Report no 5. Early vitrectomy for severe vitreous hemorrhage in diabetic retinopathy. Four-year results of a randomized trial. Arch Ophthalmol 1990; 108:958–964.
14. Aaberg TM. Pars plana vitrectomy for diabetic traction retinal detachment. Ophthalmology 1981; 88:639–642.
15. Cohen HB, McMeel JW, Franks EP. Diabetic traction detachment. Arch Ophthalmol 1979; 97:1268.
16. Charles S, Flinn CE. The natural history of diabetic extramacular traction retinal detachment. Arch Ophthalmol 1981; 99:66–68.
17. Aaberg TM. Clinical results in vitrectomy for diabetic traction retinal detachment. Am J Ophthalmol 1979; 88:246–253.
18. Rice TA, Michels RG, Rice EF. Vitrectomy for diabetic traction retinal detachment involving the macula. Am J Ophthalmol 1983; 95:22–33.
19. Meredith TA, Kaplan HJ, Aaberg TM. Pars plana vitrectomy techniques for relief of epiretinal traction by membrane segmentation. Am J Ophthalmol 1980; 89:408.
20. Charles S. VItreous microsurgery. Baltimore: Williams & Wilkins; 1981:107–120.
21. Abrams GW, Williams GA. "En bloc" excision of diabetic membranes. Am J Ophthalmol 1987; 103: 302–308.
22. Williams DF, Williams GA, Hartz A, Mieler WF, Abrams GW, Aaberg TM. Results of vitrectomy for diabetic traction retinal detachments using the en bloc excision technique. Ophthalmology 1989; 96:752–758.
23. Rice TA, Michels RG, Rice EF. Vitrectomy for diabetic rhegmatogenous retinal detachment. Am J Ophthalmol 1983; 95:34–44.
24. Thompson JT, deBustros S, Michels RG, et al. Results and prognostic factors in vitrectomy for diabetic traction–rhegmatogenous retinal detachment. Arch Ophthalmol 1987; 105:503.
25. Lewis H, Abrams GW, Foos RY. Clinicopathologic findings in anterior hyaloidal fibrovascular proliferation after diabetic vitrectomy. Am J Ophthalmol 1987; 104:614–618.
26. Lewis H, Abrams GW, Williams GA. Anterior hyaloidal fibrovascular proliferation after diabetic vitrectomy. Am J Ophthalmol 1987; 104:607–613.
27. Aaberg TM, Maggiano JM. Choroidal edema associated with retinal detachment repair. Experimental and clinical correlation. Mod Probl Ophthalmol 1979; 20:6.
28. Shea M. Early vitrectomy in proliferative diabetic retinopathy. Arch Ophthalmol 1983; 101:1204–1205.
29. O'Hanley GP, Canny CLB. Diabetic dense premacular hemorrhage. Ophthalmology 1985; 92:507–511.
30. Blankenship G. Management of vitreous cavity hemorrhage following pars plana vitrectomy for diabetic retinopathy. Ophthalmology 1986; 93:34–44.
31. Sebestyen JG. Fibrinoid syndrome: a severe compli-

cation of vitrectomy surgery in diabetics. Ann Ophthalmol 1982; 14:853–856.

32. Lewis H, Han D, Williams GA. Management of fibro-pupillary block glaucoma after pars plana vitrectomy with intravitreal gas injection. Am J Ophthalmol 1987; 103:180.

33. Lewis H, Abrams GW, Foos RY. Clinicopathologic findings in anterior hyaloidal fibrovascular proliferative after diabetic vitrectomy. Am J Ophthalmol 1987; 104:614.

34. Thompson JT, Auer CL, DeBustros S, Michels RG, Rice TA, Glaser BM. Prognostic indicators of success and failure in vitrectomy for diabetic retinopathy. Ophthalmology 1986; 93:290–295.

35. Rice TA, Michels RG, Maguire MG, Rice EF. The effect of lensectomy on the incidence of iris neovascularization and neovascular glaucoma after vitrectomy for diabetic retinopathy. Am J Ophthalmol 1983; 95:1–11.

36. Blankenship G, Cortez, R, Machemer R. The lens and pars plana vitrectomy for diabetic retinopathy complications. Arch Ophthalmol 1979; 97:1263.

37. Thompson JT, deBustros S, Michels RG, et al. Results and prognostic factors in vitrectomy for diabetic traction detachment of the macula. Arch Ophthalmol 1987; 105:497.

38. Murphy RP, Egbert PR. Regression of iris neovascularization following panretinal photocoagulation. Arch Ophthalmol 1979; 97:700.

39. DeBustros S, Thompson JT, Michels RG, Rice TA. Vitrectomy for progressive proliferative diabetic retinopathy. Arch Ophthalmol 1987; 104:196–199.

40. Liggett PE, Lean JS, Barlow WE, Ryan SJ. Intraoperative argon endophotocoagulation for recurrent vitreous hemorrhage after vitrectomy for diabetic retinopathy. Am J Ophthalmol 1987; 103:146–149.

41. Blankenship GW, Flynn HW, Kokame GT. Posterior chamber intraocular lens insertion during pars plana lensectomy and vitrectomy for complications of proliferative diabetic retinopathy. Am J Ophthalmol 1980; 108:1–5.

42. Smiddy WE, Stark WJ, Michels RG, et al. Cataract extraction after vitrectomy. Ophthalmology 1987; 94:483.

43. Hutton WL, Pesicka GA, Fuller DG. Cataract extraction in the diabetic eye after vitrectomy. Am J Ophthalmol 1987; 104:1.

Diabetic Retinopathy: Practical Management, by
R. Joseph Olk and Carol M. Lee. J.B. Lippincott Company, Philadelphia © 1993.

CHAPTER · 8

Indications for Fluorescein Angiography in the Management of Diabetic Retinopathy

Fluorescein angiography has helped in the diagnosis, management, and study of the pathophysiologic mechanisms of diabetic retinopathy. The specific indications for fluorescein angiography will be described in this chapter, underscoring the established basic guidelines outlined in the recently published *Preferred Practice Pattern* by the American Academy of Ophthalmology.[1]

NONPROLIFERATIVE DIABETIC RETINOPATHY

Fluorescein angiography is not indicated as a screening tool for diabetic retinopathy, nor as a baseline measurement of mild-to-moderate nonproliferative diabetic retinopathy. The signs of nonproliferative diabetic retinopathy should be visible on clinical examination.[2–8] Ophthalmoscopy of a well-dilated fundus performed by trained ophthalmologists and technical personnel has been shown to agree with fundus photography in at least 85% of cases; disagreement occurred in cases of the earliest stages of retinopathy whereby a photographically observable microaneurysm may not be visualized ophthalmoscopically.[9,10] The risk of underevaluating retinopathy consistently occurred in eyes with minimal changes. Clinical identification of more severe changes was almost always consistent and in agreement with the photographic findings.

Fundus stereophotography provides a permanent record of the fundus appearance and can be used to document the severity and progression of disease.[1,5,6,9–12] The seven standard fields of fundus color stereophotography, as specified by the modified Airlie House classification,[3] allows both detailed grading and documentation of progression of disease or, conversely, a response to treatment. Fundus photography is clearly valuable in documenting retinopathy that is changing rapidly, or immediately before treatment, once the decision to treat has been made on clinical grounds. Large 60° fields will give a more complete view of the midperipheral regions than 30° photography and may be the field of choice for scanning for retinopathy. Given the high specificity and sensitivity of the clinical ophthalmoscopic examination, a dilated fundus examination, possibly with fundus stereophotographs, but not fluorescein angiography, is recommended for the management of nonproliferative diabetic retinopathy.

UNEXPLAINED VISUAL LOSS

Fluorescein angiography can be helpful in determining the cause of unexplained visual loss in an eye with visual complaints out of proportion to the retinopathy clinically seen.[1,8,13,14] An eye may have both minimal peripheral changes and minimal macular edema, but visual acuity

far worse than the clinical examination indicates (Fig. 8-1). Causes may include an optic neuropathy or a markedly ischemic macula, the latter of which could be confirmed by angiography.

Occlusion of the perifoveal capillaries is readily shown on angiography[2,4,13,14] as abnormalities of the foveal avascular zone (FAZ). These angiographic characteristics include an irregularity of the margins of the FAZ, budding of capillaries into the FAZ, and the development of wide intercapillary spaces within bridging vessels in the perifoveal capillary bed.[2,13] The perifoveal capillaries may actually be more apparent owing to both dilation of the remaining capillaries and their contrast to the

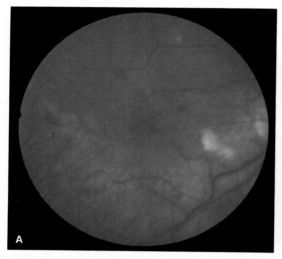

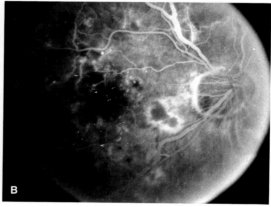

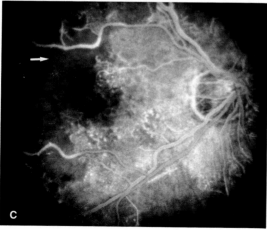

Figure 8–1 A 52-year-old white woman presented with minimal macular edema and with a history of recent vision loss. (**A**) Clinical examination showed nonproliferative retinopathy, with minimal macular edema; visual acuity was 20/50. (**B**) Fluorescein angiography revealed severe capillary nonperfusion, especially temporal to the foveal avascular zone, but no central leakage. Because there was no frank macular edema and because there were extensive areas of capillary nonperfusion, no laser photocoagulation was recommended. The patient was followed, and (**C**) the macular ischemia progressed, as seen on the fluorescein angiogram 6 years after initial presentation; visual acuity had diminished to 20/80. Note the further loss of the capillary bed, compared with (**B**) the previous fluorescein angiogram. *Comment:* This is an example of a patient with unexplained visual loss out of proportion to the clinical examination. A fluorescein angiogram is indicated.

larger zone of nonperfusion, seen angiographically as hypofluorescence. The enlargement of the FAZ is presumed to cause a loss of visual acuity from macular ischemia.[1,2,13–15]

MACULAR EDEMA

The diagnosis of clinically significant macular edema is based on examination by slit-lamp stereobiomicroscopy or fundus stereophotography.[15,16] Fluorescein angiography is not indicated to diagnose the presence of clinically significant macular edema. Angiographic evidence of fluorescein leakage, without clinical evidence of retinal thickening, does not fulfill the criteria for clinical significance. However, once the diagnosis and the decision to treat macular edema have been made, fluorescein angiography is extremely useful in helping guide the treatment pattern. Angiography will identify treatable lesions and delineate the FAZ and the status of the macular perfusion. If the fluorescein angiogram reveals marked capillary nonperfusion and it is felt that any laser treatment would critically compromise any remaining perifoveal vessels, conservative management without any intervention is indicated. Fluorescein angiography will also confirm the presence of thickening and edema by leakage in the late stage of the angiogram, which also can be used as a guide to treatment (Fig. 8-2).

Although the Early Treatment Diabetic Retinopathy Study (ETDRS) showed a treatment benefit at all levels of visual acuity, if an eye has good vision and is asymptomatic, one can elect to follow the patient, rather than treat immediately. That patient should be followed at close intervals—at least every 3 months. A fluorescein angiogram is not indicated until the decision to treat has been made based on the clinical examination (Fig. 8-3).

The ETDRS has emphasized the use of focal treatment in the treatment of diabetic macular edema characterized by focal leakage. As we have discussed, diffuse diabetic macular edema may present a different pathophysiologic mechanism. Focal edema is a product mainly of individual leaking microaneurysms, whereas diffuse diabetic macular edema may be produced by a combination of a breakdown of the inner blood–retinal barrier, at the level of the retinal capillaries and arterioles, and at the outer blood–retinal barrier, at the level of the retinal pigment epithelium.[2,17] Other treatment protocols, including Olk's modified grid photocoagulation, emphasize the use of grid treatment for diffuse macular edema greater than two disc diameters in area and involving any portion of the FAZ.[18–20] Again, the diagnosis of diffuse macular edema is made on the clinical biomicroscopic examination, whereas the fluorescein angiogram is obtained only after the decision to treat has been made and is used as a guide to treatment.

Supplemental macular treatment was required by the ETDRS if macular edema involved or threatened the center of the macula. Supplemental treatment was allowed for any degree of edema that met one of the definitions for clinical significance.[15,16,21] Fluorescein angiography is again useful in guiding the treatment, once the clinical need for retreatment has been determined. We recommend that supplemental macular photocoagulation be given if residual central thickening involving the FAZ is seen on clinical examination.[18–20] Only if retreatment is being considered does one obtain a fluorescein angiogram to delineate the areas of leakage, to identify the FAZ, and to guide in the pattern of treatment (Fig. 8-4).

PROLIFERATIVE DIABETIC RETINOPATHY

The Diabetic Retinopathy Study (DRS) has shown the clear benefit of scatter panretinal photocoagulation to certain high-risk eyes in preventing severe visual loss from the consequences of proliferative disease.[22,23] The ETDRS has recently stated that eyes with early proliferative retinopathy may benefit from early photocoagulation.[24] Fluorescein angiography is not needed to diagnose the presence of either high-risk retinopathy or early proliferative retinopathy. The clinical examination is highly sensitive in detecting this stage of retinopathy

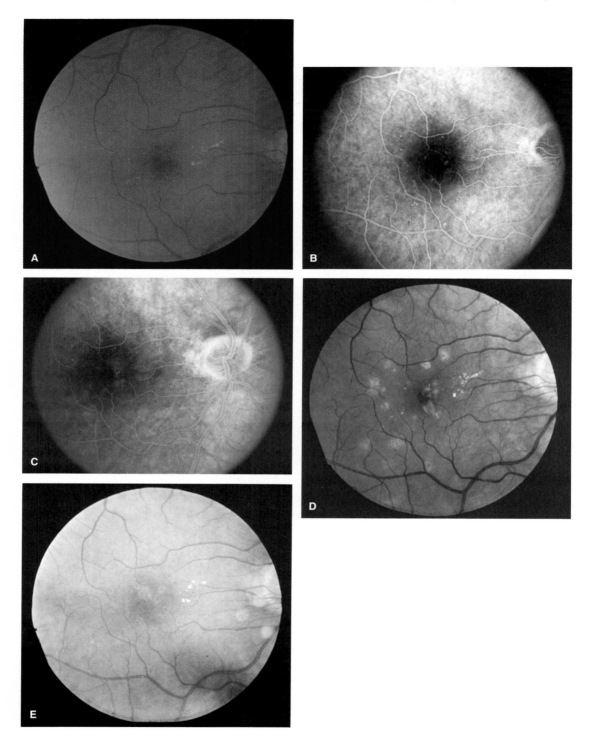

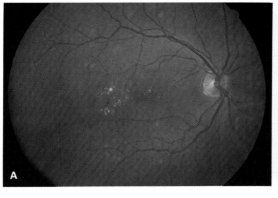

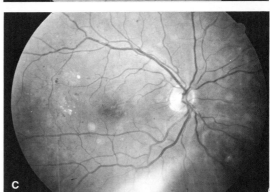

Figure 8–3 A 31-year-old man, with a 2-year history of insulin-dependent diabetes on routine annual examination, presented with (**A**) early clinically significant diabetic macular edema in his right eye. Visual acuity was 20/25 in the right eye, and it was elected to follow the patient at intervals of 3 to 4 months. (**B**) Partial spontaneous resolution of the macular thickening was noted 2 years later; (**C**) completed resolution of the macular thickening without recurrence was noted 4 years after initial presentation, with visual acuity remaining at 20/25 in his right eye. *Comment:* This case illustrates an example in which fluorescein angiography was not indicated, since the decision was made to not institute treatment and to follow the patient clinically.

and is adequate to determine the need for photocoagulation.[1,9–11] As previously stated, fundus color photography, employing the seven standard stereofields may be helpful in gauging the response to therapy, once panretinal photocoagulation has been instituted.

Because it has been shown that diabetic macular edema may be exacerbated by panretinal photocoagulation,[25–27] any eye that shows clinical evidence of retinal thickening, falling within the definition of clinically significant macular edema, should have a fluorescein angiogram to guide in the treatment of the macular edema, either before or in combination with the panretinal treatment for the proliferative disease.

Fluorescein angiography may be helpful in searching for subtle patches of neovascularization or capillary nonperfusion when either severe nonproliferative signs are present or proliferative disease is suspected, and media opacity precludes a good view. In this last cir-

◄**Figure 8–2** A 57-year-old man, with a 15-year history of noninsulin-dependent diabetes, complained of decreased vision in his right eye. Visual acuity was 20/40. (**A**) Examination revealed clinically significant macular edema by slit-lamp biomicroscopy using ETDRS criteria. Laser photocoagulation was recommended, and (**B,C**) a fluorescein angiogram was obtained. (**D**) Focal treatment was performed, and on follow-up examination 4 months later, resolution of the thickening was seen, with a visual acuity of 20/20. Because no further treatment was indicated, no further angiograms were performed. (**E**) Serial follow-up examinations showed complete resolution of his macular edema, without recurrence, and 2 years after treatment his visual acuity remained at 20/20. *Comment:* This is an example of a patient who required fluorescein angiography after the initial decision to treat his diabetic macular edema was made from clinical examination. Because on follow-up examination his clinically significant diabetic macular edema had resolved and no further treatment was indicated, no additional fluorescein angiograms were needed.

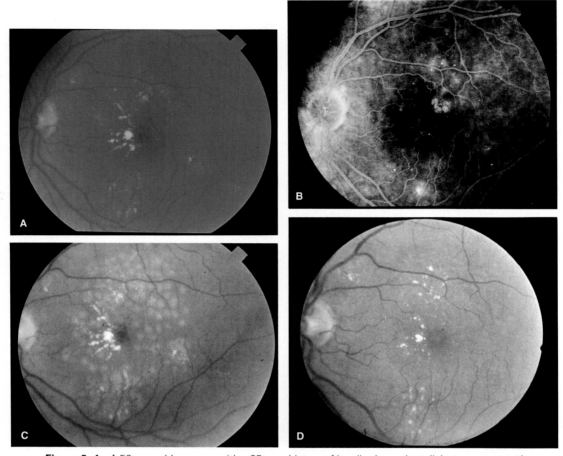

Figure 8–4 A 59-year-old woman, with a 25-year history of insulin-dependent diabetes, presented with (**A**) diffuse retinal thickening involving the foveal avascular zone, hard exudates scattered throughout the parafoveal region, and a central foveal cyst in the left eye. Visual acuity was 20/60. (**B**) Modified grid laser photocoagulation was recommended and fluorescein angiography performed. (**C**) Modified grid photocoagulation was applied to all areas of retinal thickening up to and including the edge of the foveal avascular zone. She returned for follow-up 4 months later with some reduction of her intraretinal lipid and thickening; however, (**D**) the central retinal thickening and central foveal cyst persisted. Supplemental photocoagulation was advised, and (**E**) a fluorescein angiogram was repeated. (**F**) Supplemental modified grid laser photocoagulation was applied to all areas of residual retinal thickening. Four months later she returned with (**G**) near-complete resorption of the intraretinal lipid and flattening of the central foveal avascular zone; visual acuity had improved to 20/30. Because no additional treatment was required, fluorescein angiography was not repeated. One year later visual acuity had improved to 20/20 without (**H**) evidence of any recurrence. *Comment:* This case illustrates that fluorescein angiography is indicated once the decision to treat or to do supplemental treatment has been made from clinical findings. Once the central thickening involving the foveal avascular zone has resolved and no further supplemental treatment is indicated, fluorescein angiography is no longer required.

(continued)

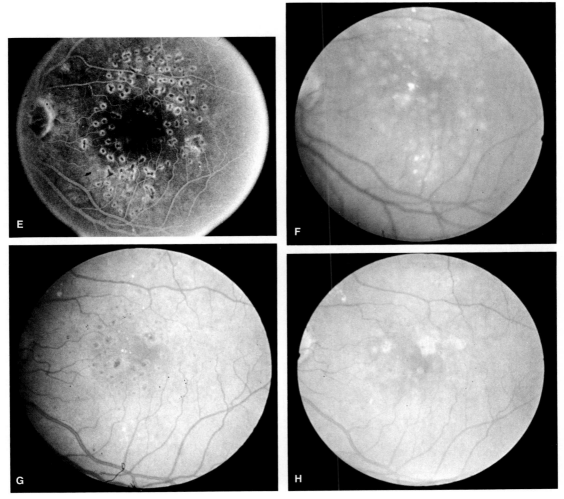

Figure 8–4 (continued)

cumstance, fluorescein angioscopy may be more helpful in scanning the retina to detect areas of leakage from neovascularization; however, fluorescein angioscopy is not helpful in the confirmation nor in the guidance of treatment for macular edema. Angiography may also be helpful in detecting specific fronds of neovascularization when blood from a vitreous hemorrhage obscures the view (Fig. 8-5). This can guide the ophthalmologist to areas of active neovascularization that may be treated with focal ablation.

In general, indications for retreatment include increasing neovascularization, new areas of neovascularization, new vitreous hemorrhage, and failure of the initial neovascularization to regress.[1,23,28] Each of these findings should be determined on clinical examination and usually do not need fluorescein angiography for confirmation. However, the progression or regression of neovascularization can be readily followed by serial clinical examinations and on fundus color photography, and can be used as a permanent record for comparison.

The significance of capillary nonperfusion in the midperipheral retina has been illustrated in the fluorescein angiographic studies by Shimizu and colleagues.[29,30] Clinically, the angio-

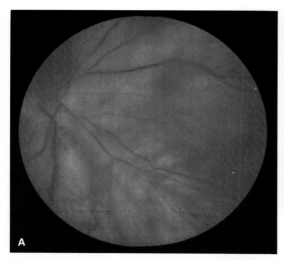

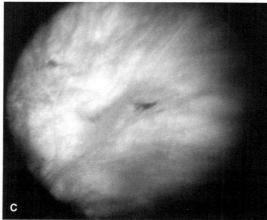

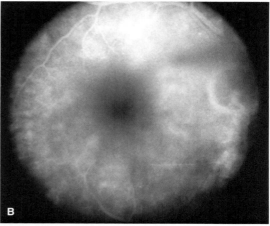

Figure 8–5 A 73-year-old white woman, with a 20-year history of insulin-dependent diabetes, presented with (**A**) central vitreous hemorrhage in her right eye. Visual acuity was 20/200. No neovascularization was seen on clinical examination; however, the view was obscured by moderate vitreous hemorrhage. Because we were concerned about the possibility of underlying occult proliferative retinopathy, fluorescein angiography was performed (**B,C**) with a *sweep of the periphery,* but we were unable to demonstrate any definite neovascularization because no leakage from occult islands of neovascularization was noted. Six weeks later, the vitreous hemorrhage spontaneously cleared and visual acuity improved to 20/20. No evidence of any proliferative disease either on the optic disc or elsewhere was noted, and it was ultimately determined that the vitreous hemorrhage occurred secondary to a posterior vitreous detachment. *Comment:* Angiography was performed here to detect any leakage consistent with neovascularization that might have been the source of vitreous hemorrhage. The retinal details were obscured clinically by the vitreous hemorrhage.

graphic demonstration of a significant amount of capillary nonperfusion or dropout may occasionally be helpful in those circumstances for which photocoagulation treatment is being considered for very severe nonproliferative or early proliferative disease.

Although the ETDRS recently showed that angiographic grading criteria can predict the progression of severe nonproliferative or early proliferative retinopathy to more advanced stages of proliferative disease, we agree with their conclusion that this finding is of no real clinical significance, since both clinical examination and fundus color photography can accurately assess the status of the eye and, since the ETDRS found that, with appropriate follow-up, eyes that were randomized to deferral of treatment had relatively low rates of severe visual loss.[31] Thus, there is no urgency or indication for angiography for earlier detection of those eyes that might progress to more advanced disease than by careful and timely clinical evaluation.

PSEUDOPHAKIC VERSUS DIABETIC MACULAR EDEMA

Fluorescein angiography may be helpful in differentiating between macular edema secondary to pseudophakia or to diabetes, as the clinical diagnosis between the two is often difficult. Typically, in pseudophakic macular edema, cysts distributed in a petalloid pattern can be appreciated by slit-lamp biomicroscopy.[32] Fluorescein angiography will usually show early dye leakage from the parafoveal capillaries in a uniform fashion with the later phases revealing a polycystic pattern of dye accumulation caused by serous exudation into the extracellular space. In addition, the capillaries of the optic nerve head will frequently leak dye in the later frames of the angiogram. Diabetic macular edema, however, is sometimes accompanied by a cystoid component, so differentiation between the two can be difficult (Fig. 8-6).

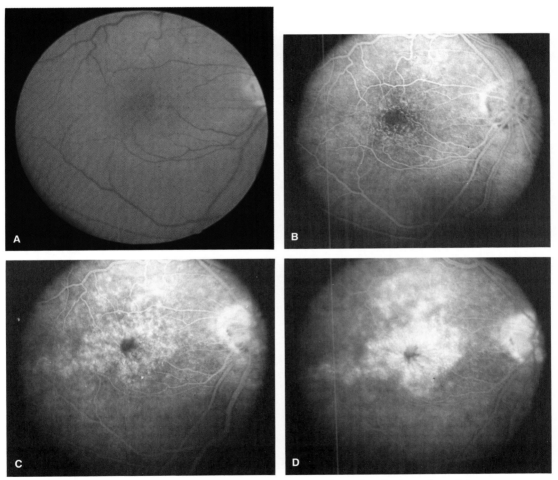

Figure 8–6 A 65-year-old woman, with a 5-year history of non–insulin-dependent diabetes, presented with visual acuity of 20/80 in her right eye 5 months after uncomplicated extracapsular cataract extraction and an intraocular lens implant. (**A**) Clinical examination revealed cystic thickening of the macula, without evidence of diabetic retinopathy. A fluorescein angiogram was obtained, which confirmed the diagnosis of pseudophakic cystoid macular edema. (**B**) The early frames of the angiogram revealed an intact foveal avascular zone; (**C**) as the study progressed, uniform diffuse leakage was noted, with (**D**) the petalloid appearance of dye accumulation seen in the latest frame. Note also the late-staining of the optic disc. *Comment:* The differential between pseudophakic or aphakic cystoid macular edema and diabetic macular edema is often difficult, despite fluorescein angiography. The angiogram shown here is characteristic of classic pseudophakic cystoid macular edema.

SUMMARY

In conclusion, fluorescein angiography is a useful guide in the treatment of clinically significant macular edema, as the means of evaluating an eye with unexplained visual loss, and sometimes in identifying subtle areas of neovascularization or capillary nonperfusion. It is not indicated for the diagnosis of either clinically significant diabetic macular edema or proliferative diabetic retinopathy. Nor is it used routinely as a screening tool or a baseline examination in patients with diabetic retinopathy.

ACKNOWLEDGMENT

This chapter has been reproduced in part from Tasman W, Jaeger EA, eds. Duane's foundations of clinical ophthalmology, vol 2, Philadelphia: JB Lippincott; 1991:1–11.

References

1. American Academy of Ophthalmology. Preferred practice pattern. Diabetic retinopathy. San Francisco: American Academy of Ophthalmology, 1989.
2. Bresnick GH. Background diabetic retinopathy. In: Ryan SJ, ed. Retina. St. Louis: CV Mosby Co; 1989:327–366.
3. Diabetic Retinopathy Study Research Group. Report no 7. A modification on the Airlie House classification of diabetic retinopathy. Invest Ophthalmol Vis Sci 1981; 212:210–226.
4. Frank RN. Etiologic mechanisms in diabetic retinopathy. In: Ryan SJ, ed. Retina. St. Louis: CV Mosby Co; 1989:30–326.
5. Javitt JC, Canner JK, Sommer A. Cost effectiveness of current approaches to the control of retinopathy in type I diabetes. Ophthalmology 1989; 96:255.
6. Javitt JC, Canner JK, Frank RG, et al. Detecting and treating retinopathy in patients with type I diabetes mellitus. Ophthalmology 1990; 97:483–495.
7. Kohner EM, Sleightholm M, Kroc Collaborative Study Group (appended). Does microaneurysm count reflect severity of early diabetic retinopathy? Ophthalmology 1986; 93:586–589.
8. Wilkinson CP. The clinical examination: limitation and over-utilization of angiographic services. Ophthalmology 1986; 93:401–404.
9. Moss SE, Klein R, Kessler SD, Richie KA. Comparison between ophthalmoscopy and fundus photography in determining severity of diabetic retinopathy. Ophthalmology 1985; 92:62–67.
10. Sussman EJ, Tsiaras WG, Soper KA. Diagnosis of diabetic eye disease. JAMA 1982; 247:3231–3234.
11. Klein BEK, Davis MD, Segal P, et al. Diabetic retinopathy. Assessment of severity and progression. Ophthalmology 1984; 91:10–17.
12. Klein R, Klein BEK, Neider NW, et al. Diabetic retinopathy as detected using ophthalmoscopy, a nonmydriate camera and standard fundus camera. Ophthalmology 1985; 92:485.
13. Bresnick GH, Condit R, Syrjala S, Palta M, Groo A, Korth K. Abnormalities of the foveal avascular zone in diabetic retinopathy. Arch Ophthalmol 1984; 102:1286–1293.
14. Bresnick GH, Engerman R, Davis MD, et al. Patterns of ischemia in diabetic retinopathy. Trans Am Acad Ophthalmol Otolaryngol 1976; 81:694.
15. Early Treatment Diabetic Retinopathy Study Research Group. Report no 1. Photocoagulation for diabetic macular edema. Arch Ophthalmol 1985; 103:1796–1806.
16. Early Treatment Diabetic Retinopathy Study Research Group. Report no 2. Treatment techniques and clinical guidelines for photocoagulation of diabetic macular edema. Ophthalmology 1987; 947:761–774.
17. Bresnick GH. Diabetic maculopathy: a critical review highlighting diffuse macular edema. Ophthalmology 1983; 90:1301–1317.
18. Olk RJ. Modified grid argon (blue-green) laser photocoagulation for diffuse diabetic macular edema. Ophthalmology 1986; 93:938–950.
19. Olk RJ. Argon green (514 nm) versus krypton red (647 nm) modified grid laser photocoagulation for diffuse diabetic macular edema. Ophthalmology 1990; 97:1101–1113.
20. Lee CM, Olk RJ. Modified grid laser photocoagulation for diffuse diabetic macular edema: long-term visual results. Ophthalmology 1991; 98:1594–1602.
21. Early Treatment Diabetic Retinopathy Study Research Group. Report no 4. Photocoagulation for diabetic macular edema. Int Ophthalmol Clin 1987; 27:265–272.
22. Diabetic Retinopathy Study Research Group. Photocoagulation treatment of proliferative diabetic retinopathy: the second report of diabetic retinopathy/vitrectomy study findings. Am J Ophthalmol 1978; 85:82–106.
23. Diabetic Retinopathy Study Research Group. Report no 14. Indication for photocoagulation treatment of diabetic retinopathy. Int Ophthalmol Clin 1987; 27:239.
24. Early Treatment Diabetic Retinopathy Study Research Group. Report no 9. Early photocoagulation for diabetic retinopathy. Ophthalmology 1991; 98:766–785.
25. McDonald HR, Schatz H. Macular edema following panretinal photocoagulation. Retina 1985; 5:5–10.
26. McDonald HR, Schatz H. Visual loss following pan-

retinal photocoagulation for proliferative diabetic retinopathy. Ophthalmology 1985; 92:388–393.

27. Meyers SM. Macular edema after scatter laser photocoagulation for proliferative diabetic retinopathy. Am J Ophthalmol 1980; 90:210–216.

28. Early Treatment Diabetic Retinopathy Study Research Group. Report no 3. Techniques for scatter and local photocoagulation treatment of diabetic retinopathy. Int Ophthalmol Clin 1987; 274:254–264.

29. Shimizu K, Kobayaski Y, Muraoka K. Midperipheral fundus involvement in diabetic retinopathy. Ophthalmology 1981; 88:601–612.

30. Niki T, Muraoka K, Shimizu K. Distribution of capillary nonperfusion in early-stage diabetic retinopathy. Ophthalmology 1984; 91:1431–1439.

31. Early Treatment Diabetic Retinopathy Study Research Group. Report no 13. Fluorescein angiographic risk factors for progression of diabetic retinopathy. Ophthalmology 1991; 98:834–840.

32. Gass JDM. Retinal capillary disease. Stereoscopic atlas of macular diseases. St Louis: CV Mosby Co; 1987:368–373.

Diabetic Retinopathy: Practical Management, by R. Joseph Olk and Carol M. Lee. J.B. Lippincott Company, Philadelphia © 1993.

CHAPTER · 9

Complications and Side Effects of Treatment

Complications of treatment can occur, although most side effects are transient and self-limited. Nevertheless, any time treatment is recommended, the patient and physician must be aware of the possible adverse side effects. We will discuss the complications associated specifically with photocoagulation in this chapter. The general complications of both anesthesia and vitrectomy surgery should be recalled, but will not be reviewed here.

ANTERIOR SEGMENT

In the anterior segment, the diabetic cornea is more susceptible to epithelial erosion and abrasion, such that a contact lens may create an iatrogenic corneal epithelial defect. Some authors have shown that a soft contact lens placed on the corneal surface before the photocoagulation session enables both safe and adequate treatment[1]; we have rarely found it necessary to do so. Theoretically argon blue-green wavelength is absorbed preferentially by the yellow pigment within nuclear sclerotic lenses, and this absorption of blue light can cause coagulation of lens proteins, with resultant nonprogressive opacities.[2,3] Currently, we use mainly the green wavelength, which does not have the same absorption spectrum as the blue wavelength, with as low-power setting as possible to achieve the appropriate intensity burn. Iris stromal burns and posterior synechiae can be avoided by careful focusing of the laser beam on the retinal tissues before each laser burn.

The posterior ciliary nerves may be damaged by transmitted heat into the suprachoroidal space,[4,5] causing accommodative insufficiency and asthenopia.[6] Patients may require plus lenses for reading and near work, although this is usually temporary. Additionally, an Adie's-like syndrome can occur with pupillary dilation, light-near dissociation, sector iris palsies, and denervation supersensitivity.[4,5] Avoidance of the horizontal meridians along the course of the long posterior ciliary nerves may reduce this complication.

INTRAOCULAR PRESSURE

Elevated intraocular pressure has been noted immediately following panretinal photocoagulation. This intraocular pressure elevation can occur suddenly and last several hours.[7] A reduced outflow facility may be measured by tonography in the presence of gonioscopically open angles. Conversely, angle closure may occur because of shallowing of the anterior chamber.[8] A transient acute spike in intraocular pressure may last up to several days, but is only rarely associated with the sequelae of synechiae.

Possible mechanisms include ciliary body swelling following alterations in the choroidal circulation caused by photocoagulation-induced venous stasis and choroidal inflammation. Edema of the ciliary body and detachment of the choroid may follow because of the collection of fluid.[8] Or, an annular and anterior rotation of the ciliary body[9] or choroidal detachment[10,11] could close the angle. Fluid might leak through the damaged ciliary vessels and choroidal vessels, increasing the vitreous volume and exacerbating the configuration toward angle closure.

Whatever the mechanism, this condition is usually self-limited; laser iridotomy is not indicated.[8] The pressure should be managed medically with topical and oral pressure-controlling medications, in addition to topical and oral steroids, to control the ciliary body swelling and choroidal detachment. The intraocular pressure will be highest approximately 1 day after photocoagulation, with a return to normal levels usually by 1 week without permanent damage. The incidence of this transient intraocular rise may be higher in eyes treated with complete panretinal photocoagulation in one session.[7,8,11,12] Also, a higher incidence of transient choroidal detachment has been noted in single-session complete panretinal scatter sessions.[13]

EXUDATIVE RETINAL DETACHMENT

A mechanism of vascular damage to the choroidal vessels by photocoagulation, similar to that causing choroidal detachment, is postulated, which results in an exudative retinal detachment. The retinal pigment epithelial (RPE)

cells, in addition to the choriocapillaris, are also damaged by the photocoagulation; their dysfunction may allow accumulation of an exudate[10,11] (Fig. 9-1).

The likelihood of both choroidal and ciliary effusions and detachments may be reduced by performing treatments in multiple sessions. We currently recommend performing scatter panretinal photocoagulation in multiple sessions, approximately 2 to 3 weeks apart, if the clinical circumstances allow such staggered timing. We and others have not noted any difference in treatment efficacy between single- and multiple-session panretinal treatment.[13]

HEMORRHAGE

During a laser procedure, hemorrhage that may occur is most likely caused by too small of a spot size at an intensity higher than needed. The use of krypton red may also be more likely to cause hemorrhage secondary to perforation of Bruch's membrane (Fig. 9-2). Direct treatment of raised neovascular fronds, either on the disc or elsewhere, is more likely to produce significant hemorrhage into the vitreous and is contraindicated. Theoretically, the heat effect of photocoagulation may also produce increased traction, if present, on neovascular vessels, causing hemorrhage during the laser treatment.

IATROGENIC CHOROIDAL NEOVASCULARIZATION

More importantly, Bruch's membrane can be punctured when using high-intensity small-spot sizes, especially in the macular region. This event may be heralded by an episode of bleeding at a laser photocoagulation site immediately after placing the burn. Choroidal neovascularization with chorioretinal anastomosis is well-described in patients treated for either diabetic macular edema[14-16] or proliferative diabetic retinopathy[17] following pre-

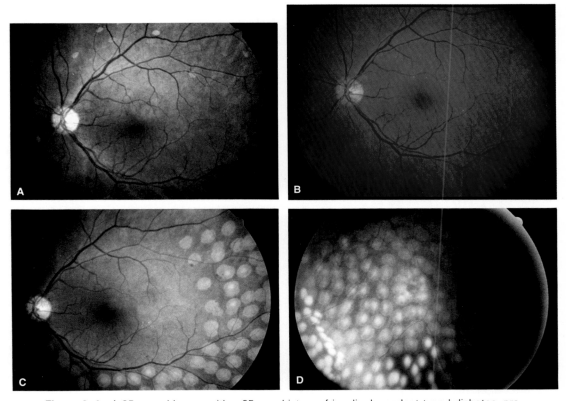

Figure 9–1 A 35-year-old man, with a 25-year history of insulin-dependent type I diabetes, presented with (**A**) nonproliferative diabetic retinopathy. Visual acuity was 20/20. He was stable over 5 years, with no changes, but then returned with (**B**) high-risk retinopathy (NVD greater than standard 10A). He received panretinal photocoagulation in two sessions, with a total of 1700 burns using the argon laser. (**C–E**) The pattern of inferior panretinal photocoagulation is shown. This was followed 3 weeks later by completion of the panretinal photocoagulation (**F,G**) to the superior one-half of the retina. The patient had regression of his NVD, and visual acuity returned to 20/25; however, (**H**) 6 months later he developed recurrent NVD with some vitreous hemorrhage. (**I**) Over the next month, he received two sessions of supplemental panretinal photocoagulation for a total of 1500 burns. Visual acuity was 20/40. Two days after supplemental treatment, he complained of decreased vision and pain. His vision had decreased to hand motions, and repeat evaluation (**K**) showed marked exudative reaction with an exudative detachment in the posterior pole (*arrow*), with (**L**) choroidal detachment peripherally (*arrow*). He was treated with topical steroids and cycloplegics, and his visual acuity improved to 20/80 over the next several weeks. (**M**) The macular exudative detachment was almost completely resolved. He was followed over the next 3 years with (**N**) regression of his proliferative disease and no recurrence of the macular edema. Visual acuity returned to 20/40.

(continued)

sumed iatrogenic breaks in Bruch's membrane with both the argon green and krypton red laser wavelengths. Specific breaks, however, may not be needed. Choriocapillaris endothelial budding and disruption of the integrity of Bruch's membrane may be induced simply by photocoagulation, without a clinically evident break.[18] If a choroidal neovascular membrane occurs, laser photocoagulation may be effective in maintaining visual acuity,[14] but usually results in a poor visual outcome.[15,16] To avoid this unfavorable complication, we recommend the least intensity needed to achieve a light-gray burn in the macular area, a spot size larger than 50 μm, and avoidance of repeated laser burns to a single microaneurysm.

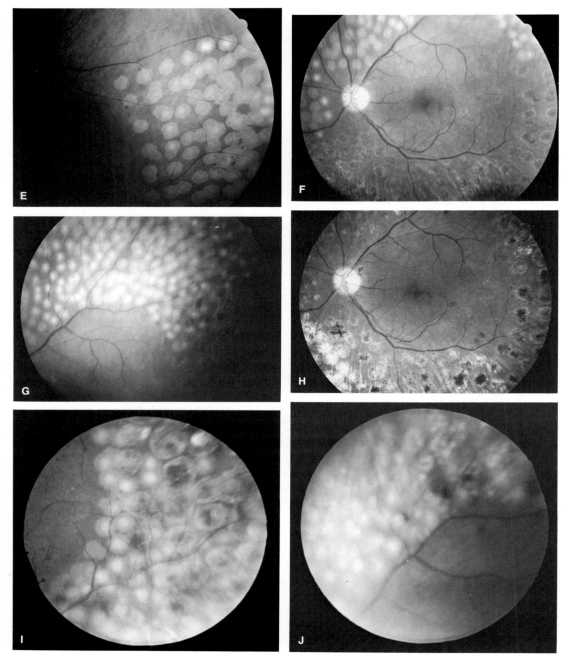

Figure 9–1 (continued)

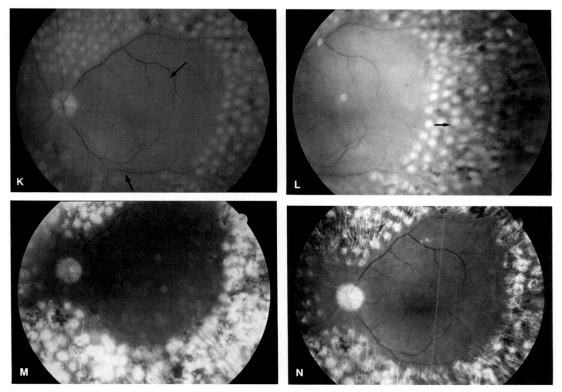

Figure 9–1 (continued)

Early recognition of a choroidal neovascular membrane is important for the eventual outcome of the eye. This complication should be suspected if a deep subretinal greenish or grayish lesion is present or if subneurosensory retinal fluid is seen, as if the edema and lipid appear to be increasing after macular photocoagulation. These signs are often quite difficult to differentiate from the normal clinical picture following uncomplicated macular photocoagulation. If a hemorrhage occurs intraoperatively, mild pressure is applied to the globe by the contact lens; this generally stops the bleeding. Direct photocoagulation of the bleeding spot with a larger-spot size of longer duration with green or yellow dye wavelength is rarely needed to stop the bleeding. We do not know if laser photocoagulation is effective in the management of iatrogenic choroidal neovascular membranes, but may be helpful in select cases.

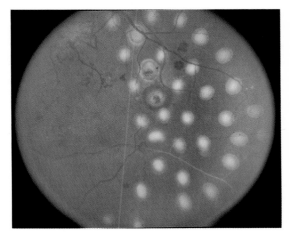

Figure 9–2 During photocoagulation with krypton red, Bruch's membrane was punctured and intraretinal hemorrhage occurred; the energy used was too high in this situation.

EPIRETINAL FIBROSIS

Epiretinal fibrosis is sometimes an unusual visually significant sequela of macular treatment; avoidance of both overly intense treatment and direct treatment of intraretinal hemorrhage may minimize this risk. Unless it is felt that the epiretinal membrane is a significant cause of visual impairment, other causes of visual loss, such as macular ischemia, should be investigated before consideration of vitrectomy and membrane peeling.

MACULAR EDEMA

Macular edema may follow panretinal photocoagulation, especially if the proliferative disease is accompanied by preexisting macular edema.[19–25] This will be discussed more completely in Chapter 10. For treatment of both macular edema and peripheral proliferative retinopathy, we recommend concurrent treatment with combined macular and panretinal photocoagulation to the inferior one-half of the retina in the first session, followed 2 to 3 weeks later by completion of the panretinal treatment in the second session.[26] This combined treatment may avoid the transient loss in vision attributed to the exacerbation of macular edema following panretinal scatter photocoagulation. Other causes of transient visual loss following panretinal photocoagulation include choroidal detachment and exudative macular detachment[13,25]; the visual loss may be mild or even severe to "light perception" or even transient "no light perception" vision.[25]

OPTIC NEUROPATHY

Rare but reported cases of severe, permanent visual loss have been attributed to thermal optic neuropathy secondary to photocoagulation burns being placed too close to the optic nerve head.[27] The photocoagulation burns may undergo lateral thermal expansion, with subsequent damage to the nerve fiber layer entering the optic nerve, in addition to damage to peripapillary choroidal and retinal vessels. We recommend treating no closer than one disc diameter from the optic nerve head and never treating neovascularization on the disc directly.

VISUAL FIELDS

Less severe and more common irreversible changes include a decrease in the peripheral visual field, more pronounced with xenon arc than with argon laser, as demonstrated in the Diabetic Retinopathy Study (DRS).[28–30] In the DRS, the peripheral field loss experienced by some patients treated with argon laser, when compared with untreated controls, was not considered statistically significant. The preliminary studies, however, are no longer directly applicable, because we do not treat neovascularization of the disc directly. Also, the perimetry performed in the DRS studies used a bright IV-4 target of the Goldmann perimeter such that the field losses reported are most likely minimized. The DRS found that approximately 25% of xenon-treated eyes suffered a modest peripheral field loss from 30° to 45° per meridian and another 25% of xenon-treated eyes suffered a peripheral loss to less than 30° per meridian. On the other hand, only 5% of argon-treated eyes experienced a field loss from 30° to 45° per meridian of peripheral visual field.[29] This small figure associated with the argon laser may again be minimized, since more sensitive testing, for instance, with a smaller test object, was not performed.

The Early Treatment Diabetic Retinopathy Study (ETDRS) recently reported its findings on the treatment of early proliferative and moderate-to-severe nonproliferative retinopathy.[20] This study found that early scatter photocoagulation, especially a more complete full pattern, gave a modest statistically significant peripheral visual field loss to Goldmann targets I-2e and I-4e, when compared with eyes serving as untreated controls.[20] Loss of peripheral visual field is more likely to occur following extensive confluent photocoagulation treatment;

furthermore, repeat treatment to areas already lasered may increase the risk of nerve fiber layer damage, resulting in greater peripheral field constriction[31] (Fig. 9-3).

Peripheral visual field loss is expected in up to 50% of eyes when careful perimetry is performed with a smaller I-4e isopter target when compared with a larger IV-4e target, as in the study by Doft and Blankenship, despite using argon treatment.[13] Following panretinal photocoagulation, up to one-half of patients may have some complaint reflecting peripheral field difficulties.[32] Theoretically, krypton red should produce less nerve fiber layer damage and thus less peripheral field loss, but studies have not shown this to be significant clinically relative to the peripheral field effects,[33] when compared with the field defects following argon wavelengths.

No difference in the effects on the central visual field could be attributed to the use of argon green versus krypton red in a recent comparative study between the two wavelengths for macular photocoagulation.[34] Annoying paracentral scotomas were common, however, earlier in the course of the study when argon blue-green was used to deliver modified grid macular treatments.[35] Paracentral scotomas, which may occur within the central 10° of eyes with untreated macular edema, are further depressed by 3 to 4 dB per treatment session when tested with automated static threshold perimetry, regardless of the wavelength used for macular photocoagulation[36] (Fig. 9-4). The initial one or two treatments of modified grid were subjectively well-tolerated in Striph and coworkers' study,[36] whereas further treatments, which are frequently clinically necessary, were seen to cause subjective loss of central light sensitivity and complaints of subjective darkening of the central field. However, because the retina within the foveal avascular zone of the macula is not treated, threshold sensitivity at fixation is maintained, despite the reduction of paracentral sensitivity.

The ETDRS has also demonstrated mild paracentral visual field defects to the I-2 test object; these were statistically insignificant when compared with untreated controls. This side effect should not be a deterrent to treatment when clinically indicated. In an attempt to reduce the frequency of these paracentral scotomas, blue-green wavelength is no longer used in macular treatments because the preferential uptake by the nerve fiber layer of the blue-green wavelength could account for more central field defects.

OTHER PSYCHOPHYSICAL FUNCTIONS

Psychophysical parameters, including loss of hue discrimination and a tritan blue-yellow defect, often present in diabetic patients, may be exacerbated by macular and panretinal photocoagulation.[32–37] Also, dark adaptation has been shown to be slower in diabetic eyes than in nondiabetic eyes. Further slowing of the dark adaptation curve occurs following panretinal photocoagulation.[38] In the study by Pender and associates,[38] after panretinal photocoagulation, the final rod threshold was 1.1 log units greater than it was before photocoagulation. Clinically, this is equivalent to the need for a light ten times brighter than normal for visual perception. In circumstances of dim-to-dark background light, such as dusk, this is visually significant. Diabetic patients frequently complain of difficulty with night vision,[32] especially when driving. This common complaint will frequently be exacerbated after treatment, and patients should be informed about these potential problems and changes incurred on their life-styles.

ENLARGEMENT OF PHOTOCOAGULATION SCAR

We have noted clinically an enlargement of the photocoagulation scar followed by permanent scarring in a rare number of our cases treated for diabetic macular edema. The enlargement or creeping of the photocoagulation scar is more typically seen, however, in eyes treated with laser photocoagulation for choroidal neovascular membranes and is more common in

(continued on page 153)

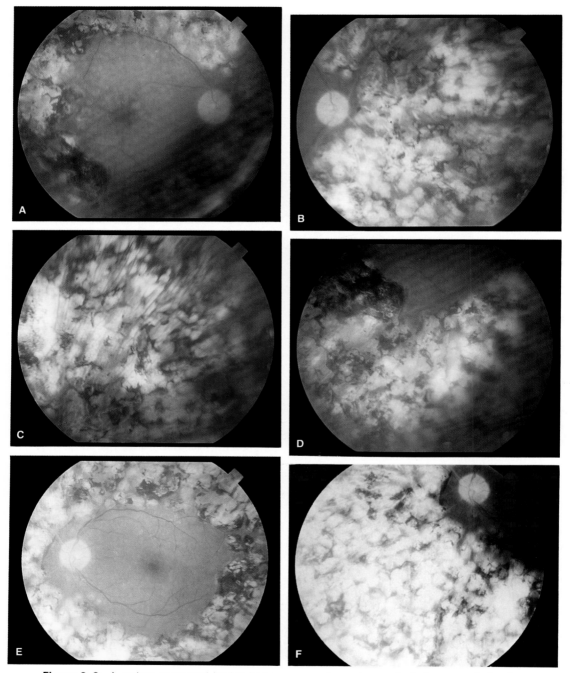

Figure 9–3 A patient presented having had seven sessions of panretinal photocoagulation for proliferative disease, resulting in (**A–H**) extensive photocoagulation scars throughout the entire fundus of both eyes. (**A,B,E**) There is mild optic pallor of both discs, with (**I,J**) marked peripheral field restriction. Central visual acuity has been maintained at 20/50.

(continued)

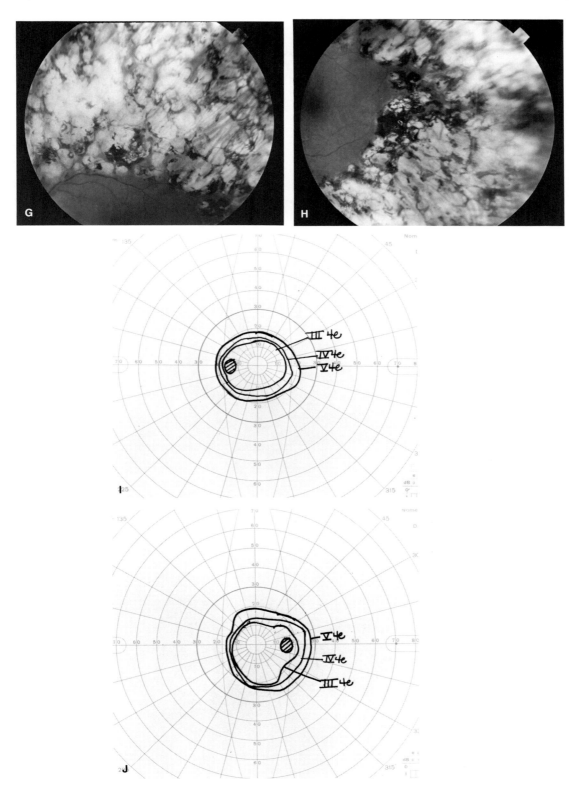

Figure 9–3 (continued)

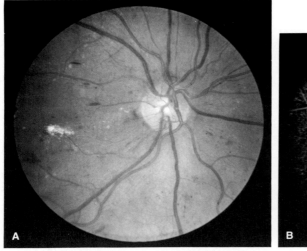

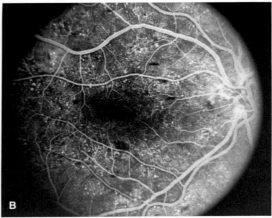

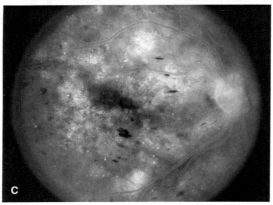

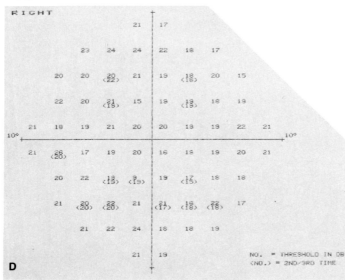

Figure 9–4 A 39-year-old white woman, with type II diabetes of 12-years duration, presented with (**A–C**) NVD and diffuse diabetic macular edema. Visual acuity was 20/25. (**D**) Preoperative Humphrey visual fields mapping macular function were within normal limits. (**E,F**) She underwent combined modified grid and panretinal photocoagulation treatment. (**G–I**) Her proliferative disease regressed, but she had persistent diabetic macular edema and cystoid macular edema and (**J**) underwent supplemental grid treatment. Four months later, (**K–M**) her central macula was flat, without evidence of thickening. However, she complained of spots in her central vision. (**N**) Repeat Humphrey visual fields confirmed several new paracentral scotomas, but her vision remained stable and visual acuity was 20/25. (**O,P**) After 2 years, there was no evidence of proliferative disease or recurrence of macular edema, but her complaint of paracentral scotomas persists.

(continued)

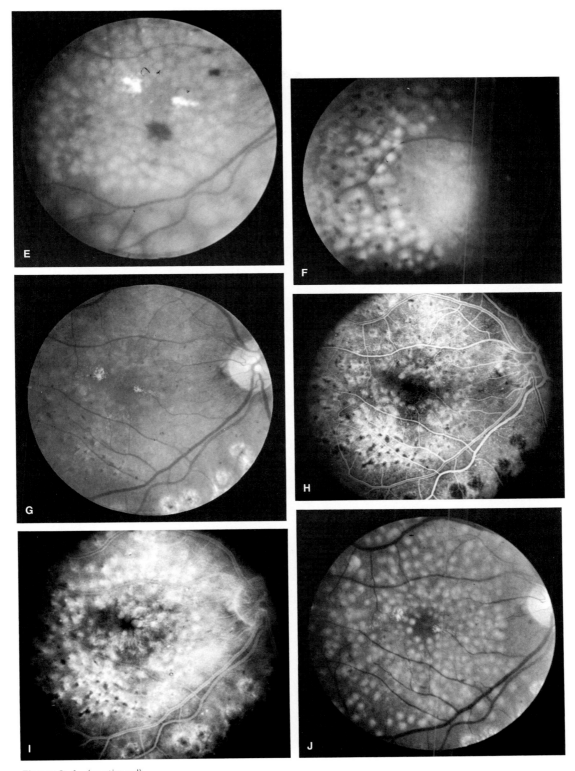

Figure 9–4 (continued)

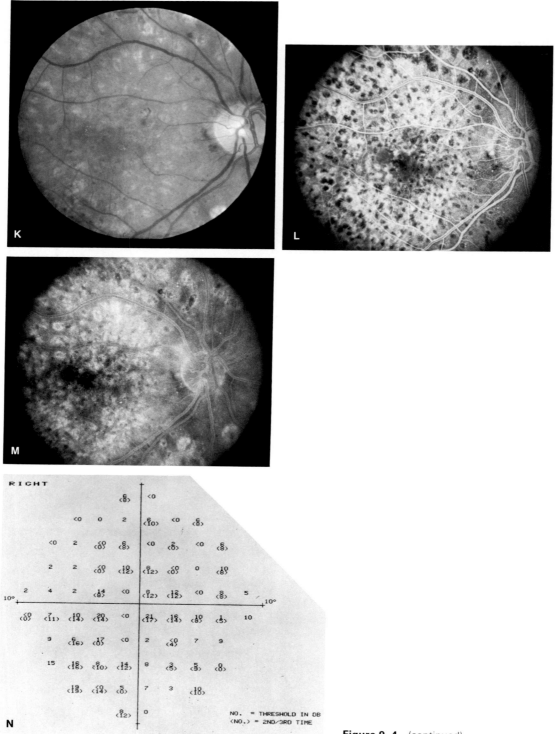

Figure 9–4 (continued)

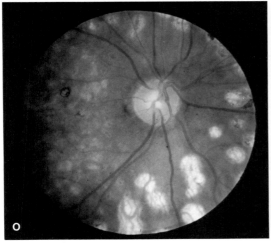

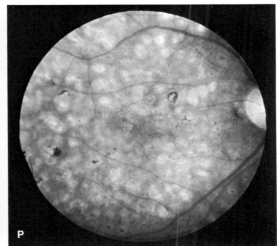

Figure 9–4 (continued)

eyes treated with the krypton red wavelength. In a recent retrospective review of eyes treated for diffuse diabetic macular edema with grid photocoagulation by Schatz and associates, 5% of the studied eyes demonstrated a progressive enlargement of the photocoagulation scars, resulting in RPE atrophy and visual loss.[39] In our experience, we have found that this "RPE creep" is only rarely associated with significant visual loss.

SUBRETINAL FIBROSIS

Subretinal fibrosis is also seen following laser photocoagulation to the macula for diabetic macular edema. We have found that this, too, occurs rarely and, in our experience, is usually seen in cases of severe, long-standing, and chronic diabetic macular edema (Fig. 9-5).

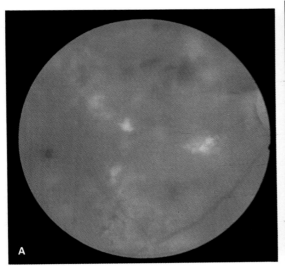

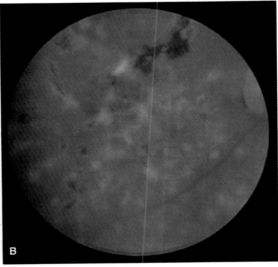

Figure 9–5 (**A**) This 65-year-old man had chronic diabetic macular edema, with thick lipid exudate and RPE hyperplasia. Two years following multiple sessions of modified grid photocoagulation the edema had resolved, but note (**B**) there is a large amount of subretinal fibrosis.

FOVEOLAR BURN

The most devastating complication of panretinal photocoagulation is an inadvertent foveolar burn. This can be avoided by meticulous observation of the topography of the eye; remember that the Rodenstock and Volk panfunduscopic lenses and Mainster posterior pole lenses are inverted images. Always locate the macula before and during treatment. When treating the macular area, a recent fluorescein angiogram should be projected either at the side of the laser with a desktop viewer or projected along the wall for following the landmarks of the macular vasculature.

When performing panretinal treatment, demarcate the temporal boundary along the macular side with three to four rows of laser burns. This serves as the temporal border along with the superotemporal and inferotemporal arcades through which centrally the photocoagulation burns should not pass. Also, peripheral treatment should be performed from posterior to anterior peripherally. When using the Goldmann three-mirror contact lens, remember to locate the macula with the central lens. When treating peripheral retina, use the peripheral mirror, positioned at 180° from the actual area being treated. Always remember whether the central lens or the mirrors are being used. If the patient is uncooperative or is mobile during laser treatment or does not understand the surgeon's instructions, retrobulbar or peribulbar anesthetic is indicated. The anesthetic risks of perforation of the globe, retrobulbar hemorrhage, central retinal artery or vein occlusion, or even respiratory arrest should be discussed before the installation of the retrobulbar or peribulbar anesthetic.

References

1. Arentsen JJ, Tasman W. Using a bandage contact lens to prevent recurrent corneal erosion during photocoagulation in patients with diabetes. Am J Ophthalmol 1981; 92:714–716.
2. Mainster MA. Wavelength selection in macular photocoagulation: tissue optics, thermal effects, and laser systems. Ophthalmology 1986; 93:952–958.
3. McCanna P, Chandra SR, Stevens TS, et al. Argon laser-induced cataract as a complication of retinal photocoagulation. Arch Ophthalmol 1982; 100:1071–1073.
4. Rogell GD. Internal ophthalmoplegia after argon laser panretinal photocoagulation. Arch Ophthalmol 1979; 97:904–905.
5. Lobes LA, Bourgnon P. Pupillary abnormalities following argon laser ablation for proliferative diabetic retinopathy. Ophthalmology 1985; 92:234–236.
6. Lerner BC, Lakhanpal V, Schocket SS. Transient myopia and accommodative paresis following cryotherapy and panretinal photocoagulation. Am J Ophthalmol 1984; 97:704–708.
7. Blondeau P, Pavan PR, Phelps CD. Acute pressure elevation following panretinal photocoagulation. Arch Ophthalmol 1981; 99:1239–1242.
8. Mensher JH. Anterior chamber depth alteration after retinal photocoagulation. Arch Ophthalmol 1977; 95:113–116.
9. Phelps C. Angle closure glaucoma secondary to ciliary body swelling. Arch Ophthalmol 1974; 92:287–290.
10. Boulton PE. A study of the mechanism of transient myopia following extensive xenon arc photocoagulation. Trans Ophthalmol Soc UK 1974; 93:287–300.
11. Huamonte FU, Peyman GA, Goldberg MF, et al. Immediate fundus complications after retinal scatter photocoagulation. I. Clinical picture and pathogenesis. Ophthalmol Surg 1976; 7:88–99.
12. Liang JC, Huamonte FU. Reduction of immediate complications after panretinal photocoagulation. Retina 1984; 4:166–170.
13. Doft BH, Blankenship GW. Single versus multiple treatment sessions of argon laser panretinal photocoagulation for proliferative diabetic retinopathy. Ophthalmology 1982; 89:772–779.
14. Varley MP, Frank E, Purnell EW. Subretinal neovascularization after focal argon laser for diabetic macular edema. Ophthalmology 1988; 95:567–573.
15. Berger AR, Boniuk I. Bilateral subretinal neovascularization after focal laser photocoagulation for diabetic macular edema. Am J Ophthalmol 1989; 108:88–90.
16. Lewis H, Schachat AP, Haimann MH, et al. Choroidal neovascularization after laser photocoagulation for diabetic macular edema. Ophthalmology 1990; 97:503–511.
17. Wallow I. Chorioretinal and choriovitreal neovascularization after photocoagulation for proliferative diabetic retinopathy. Ophthalmology 1985; 92:523–532.
18. Pollack A, Heriot WJ, Henkind P. Cellular processes causing defects in Bruch's membrane following krypton laser photocoagulation. Ophthalmology 1986; 93:1113–1119.
19. Ferris FL, Podgor MJ, Davis MD. The Diabetic Retinopathy Study Research Group. Report no 12. Macular edema in diabetic retinopathy study patients. Ophthalmology 1987; 94:754–760.

20. Early Treatment Diabetic Retinopathy Study Research Group. Report no 9. Early photocoagulation for diabetic retinopathy. Ophthalmology 1991; 98: 766–785.

21. Blankenship GW. A clinical comparison of central and peripheral argon laser panretinal photocoagulation for proliferative diabetic retinopathy. Ophthalmology 1988; 95:170–177.

22. McDonald HR, Schatz H. Visual loss following panretinal photocoagulation for proliferative diabetic retinopathy. Ophthalmology 1985; 92:388–393.

23. McDonald HR, Schatz H. Macular edema following panretinal photocoagulation. Retina 1985; 5:5–10.

24. Meyers SM. Macular edema after scatter laser photocoagulation for proliferative diabetic retinopathy. Am J Ophthalmol 1980; 90:210–216.

25. Kleiner RC, Elman MJ, Murphy RP, Ferris FL III. Transient severe visual loss after panretinal photocoagulation. Am J Ophthalmol 1988; 106:298–306.

26. Lee CM, Olk RJ. Combined modified grid and panretinal photocoagulation for diffuse diabetic macular edema and proliferative retinopathy. Presented at the 1991 meeting of the Am Acad of Ophthalmol (submitted for publication).

27. Swartz M, Apple DJ, Creel D. Sudden severe visual loss associated with peripapillary burns during panretinal argon photocoagulation. Br J Ophthalmol 1983; 67:517–519.

28. Diabetic Retinopathy Study Research Group. Photocoagulation treatment of proliferative diabetic retinopathy: the second report of diabetic retinopathy/vitrectomy study findings. Am J Ophthalmol 1978; 85:82–106.

29. Diabetic Retinopathy Study Research Group. Report no 8. Photocoagulation of proliferative diabetic retinopathy: clinical applications of DRS findings. Invest Ophthalmol Vis Sci 1981; 88:583–600.

30. Diabetic Retinopathy Study Research Group. Report no 14. Indications for photocoagulation treatment of diabetic retinopathy. Int Ophthalmol Clin 1987; 27:239–252.

31. Frank RN. Visual fields and electroretinography following extensive photocoagulation. Arch Ophthalmol 1975; 93:591–598.

32. Russel PW, Sekuler R, Fetkenhour C. Visual function after panretinal photocoagulation: a survey. Diabetes Care 1985; 8:57–63.

33. Schulenberg WE, Hamilton AM, Blach RK. A comparative study of argon laser and krypton laser in the treatment of diabetic optic disc neovascularization. Br J Ophthalmol 1979; 63:412–417.

34. Olk RJ. Argon green (514 nm) versus krypton red (647 nm) modified grid laser photocoagulation for diffuse diabetic macular edema. Ophthalmology 1990; 97:1101–1113.

35. Olk RJ. Modified grid argon (blue-green) laser photocoagulation for diffuse diabetic macular edema. Ophthalmology 1986; 93:938–950.

36. Striph GG, Hart WM, Olk RJ. Modified grid laser photocoagulation for diabetic macular edema. The effect on the central visual field. Ophthalmology 1988; 95:1673–1679.

37. Birch-Cox J. Defective colour vision in diabetic retinopathy before and after laser photocoagulation. Mod Probl Ophthalmol 1978; 19:326–329.

38. Pender PM, Benson WE, Compton H, Cox GB. The effects of panretinal photocoagulation on dark adaptation in diabetics with proliferative retinopathy. Am Acad Ophthalmol 1981; 88:635–638.

39. Schatz H, Madeira D, McDonald HR, et al. Progressive enlargement of laser scars following grid laser photocoagulation for diffuse diabetic macular edema. Arch Ophthalmol 1991; 109:1549–1551.

Diabetic Retinopathy: Practical Management, by R. Joseph Olk and Carol M. Lee. J.B. Lippincott Company, Philadelphia © 1993.

CHAPTER · 10

Special Cases

DIABETIC RETINOPATHY AND CATARACTS

Cataracts are a leading cause of reversible visual loss in the United States, whereas diabetic retinopathy is the leading cause of new blindness in working-aged (25 to 74 years) persons.[1,2] The Wisconsin Epidemiologic Study of Diabetic Retinopathy (WESDR) has shown that the severity and prevalence of diabetic retinopathy is directly correlated with the duration of diabetes.[3-7] In addition, macular edema is found more frequently in older-onset patients during the first few years after diagnosis of their systemic diabetes and is present more frequently in older-onset persons with concurrent nonproliferative diabetic retinopathy.[8,9] Because there is a high correlation between duration of diabetes and age, older patients who are more likely to have cataracts are also more likely to have retinopathy or macular edema.

In the preoperative evaluation of a patient with diabetes and cataracts, careful attention should be given to the gonioscopic evaluation and the dilated fundus examination. The state of the cornea should be checked, as it is prone to epithelial erosion. The angle must be examined, looking for early rubeosis. The macula should be examined with slit-lamp biomicroscopy, and the retinal periphery and midperiphery should be carefully examined for early neovascularization. All patients contemplating cataract surgery should have a dilated peripheral examination with the aid of scleral indentation to look for vitreoretinal lesions, including occult retinal tears. Eyes with either clinically significant diabetic macular edema or high-risk retinopathy should be considered for prompt photocoagulation before cataract surgery if visualization through the cataractous lens is possible. In patients for whom photocoagulation is precluded by the lens opacity, close postoperative follow-up is essential with photocoagulation delivered as soon as the healing of the surgical incision allows. Eyes with early macular edema should be watched carefully postoperatively, since it is our impression that underlying macular edema is exacerbated after cataract surgery. In addition, it is often difficult to distinguish between diabetic macular edema and pseudophakic macular edema of the Irvine–Gass type[10] (see following section).

Numerous reports have shown that the incidence of neovascular glaucoma and rubeosis is statistically associated with intracapsular cataract extraction,[11,12] aphakia,[13,14] and lensectomy.[15] Intracapsular cataract extraction, without regard to preoperative status of the retinopathy, was associated with an almost 8%

incidence of rubeosis or neovascular glaucoma in 1 year, and in eyes with preoperative proliferative disease, 40% of eyes developed rubeosis or neovascular glaucoma in 1 year.[11] In contrast, another study showed that none of 53 diabetic eyes undergoing extracapsular cataract extraction with maintenance of an intact posterior capsule developed rubeosis or neovascular glaucoma; however, 2 of 17 eyes developed neovascular glaucoma after extracapsular cataract extraction accompanied by primary capsulotomy.[12] Lens removal or lensectomy at the time of vitrectomy was associated with a three- to fourfold increase in postoperative rubeosis and neovascular glaucoma in Rice's review.[15] It is postulated that the loss of the posterior capsule allows the free diffusion of an angiogenic factor to reach the anterior chamber and to stimulate iris neovascularization.

We have noted clinically that some patients develop progressive retinopathy following cataract extraction with primary capsulotomy and following secondary yttrium–aluminum–garnet (YAG) laser capsulotomy. Extracapsular cataract extraction with maintenance of the posterior capsule may also be followed by progressive retinopathy. For eyes with very severe nonproliferative or early proliferative retinopathy, we recommend panretinal photocoagulation before cataract surgery or before secondary YAG capsulotomy, if possible. Cataract extraction should be performed with either an extracapsular or phacoemulsification-type technique, with all attempts at maintaining an intact posterior capsule. We generally do not recommend anterior chamber implants because of possible interference with the visualization of the iris when looking for rubeosis in the future or the additional difficulties in performing photocoagulation if needed later. Also, the angle structures may be compromised by the anterior chamber implant if the anterior segment becomes involved by neovascularization, with further compromise of the filtration apparatus.

The decision to perform cataract surgery in a patient who is diabetic relies on the generally accepted determinants of visual disability. Sometimes a cataract may not be visually disabling, but rather, is dense enough to preclude an adequate view for either diagnosis or treatment. Cataract extraction, then, is recommended for both diagnostic and therapeutic reasons. Follow-up with serial dilated examinations postoperatively should always be performed at close intervals, with photocoagulation given if indicated.

Occasionally, an eye requiring vitrectomy for the complications of proliferative retinopathy will also have a visually significant cataract. Standard cataract extraction and intraocular lens (IOL) implantation through a sclerocorneal incision can be followed during the same operation with vitrectomy. Another technique described recently involves vitrectomy with lensectomy, capsulotomy, sulcus-based or sclerally sutured posterior chamber implant, and intraoperative endolaser.[16] We have found that both techniques allow adequate intra- and postoperative visualization and treatment of the diabetic retinopathy.

MACULAR EDEMA: DIABETIC OR PSEUDOPHAKIC?

As mentioned earlier, pseudophakic cystoid macular edema often can be demonstrated angiographically following cataract extraction, but is symptomatic in far fewer cases.[10,17,18] Following uncomplicated intracapsular cataract extraction, subclinical, but angiographically evident, cystoid macular edema can be seen in up to 70% of cases in the first 2 to 3 months postoperatively, but only 5% to 15% of patients will experience visual loss.[10] Clinically, we have noted that patients with previously untreated diabetic macular edema will frequently suffer an exacerbation of their macular edema after uncomplicated cataract extraction and IOL implantation. Often the macular edema will appear cystic, and it can be difficult to distinguish, by clinical examination alone, whether the macular edema is primarily diabetic in etiology or of the Irvine–Gass type.

Here fluorescein angiography can be helpful. In pseudophakic cystoid macular edema, early uniform leakage of the perifoveal capillary bed is typically seen, with late leakage in a petalloid pattern. This is often accompanied by leakage of dye from the optic nerve head. In diabetic macular edema, either focal leakage from leaking microaneurysms or diffuse leakage from a diffusely diseased capillary bed can be seen; in this latter instance, the leakage will not generally appear as uniform. Although a polycystic pattern of leakage can be seen late in the angiogram in diffuse diabetic macular edema, it will be accompanied by a more diffuse area of leakage. Also, the optic nerve head

should not leak fluorescein, unless there is neovascularization of the disc. Because of the coexistence of cystoid macular edema with diabetic macular edema, it may be difficult to differentiate between the two causes, even with angiography (Figs. 10-1 through 10-3).

In patients in whom the cause of postoperative macular edema is clearly diabetic in origin, we recommend laser photocoagulation if clinically indicated. In patients for whom the edema appears mainly pseudophakic, we gen-

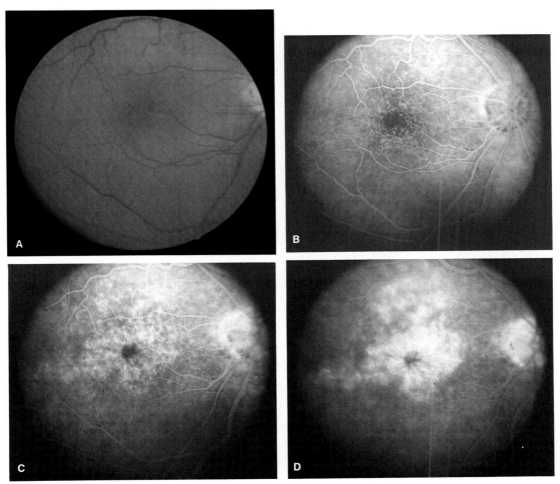

Figure 10–1 A 65-year-old woman with a 5-year history of non–insulin-dependent diabetes, presented with visual acuity of 20/80 in her right eye 5 months after an uncomplicated extracapsular cataract extraction and intraocular lens implant. (**A**) Clinical examination revealed cystic thickening of the macula, without evidence of diabetic retinopathy. A fluorescein angiogram was obtained, which confirmed the diagnosis of pseudophakic cystoid macular edema. (**B**) The early frames of the angiogram revealed an intact foveal avascular zone; (**C**) as the study progressed, uniform diffuse leakage was noted, with (**D**) the petalloid appearance of dye accumulation seen in the latest frame. Note also the late staining of the optic disc.

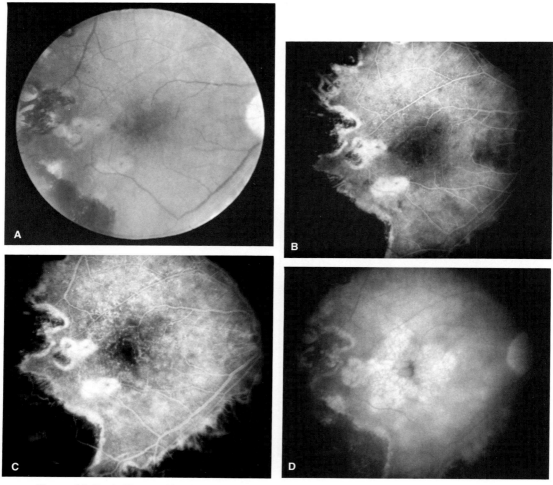

Figure 10–2 A 45-year-old white man with a history of panretinal photocoagulation presented with painless loss of vision after cataract surgery. (**A**) Fundus photography showed macular thickening with cystoid changes, and fluorescein angiography revealed diabetic macular edema with cystoid macular edema noted in the late frames. (**B–D**) The early frames show discrete areas of microaneurysm formation and irregular parafoveal capillary abnormalities, which leak late, in a cystoid and diffuse pattern. Note there is no uniform filling in the early frames, which would be more consistent with primarily pseudophakic macular edema. (**E**) The patient received modified grid laser photocoagulation for diabetic macular edema with a cystoid component. The patient had resolution of his macular edema until 1 year posttreatment when (**F,G**) he had recurrent macular edema with diffuse leakage centrally. This case demonstrates that fluorescein angiography is helpful in differentiating between primarily pseudophakic versus primarily diabetic macular edema. In this patient, the macular edema was believed to more likely represent diabetic changes, rather than pseudophakic changes and, therefore, modified grid laser photocoagulation was recommended as the initial management.

(continued)

erally follow the patient for approximately 6 months, as usually the edema will resolve spontaneously. If by 6 months the edema is still present, we will institute pharmacologic methods to try to theoretically reduce the edema. In patients for whom the cause is not clear-cut and in whom both mechanisms appear to contribute to the edema, we will try pharmacologic agents for 4 to 6 months; if then there is still persistence of the edema, we consider macular photocoagulation in an effort to reduce the edema.

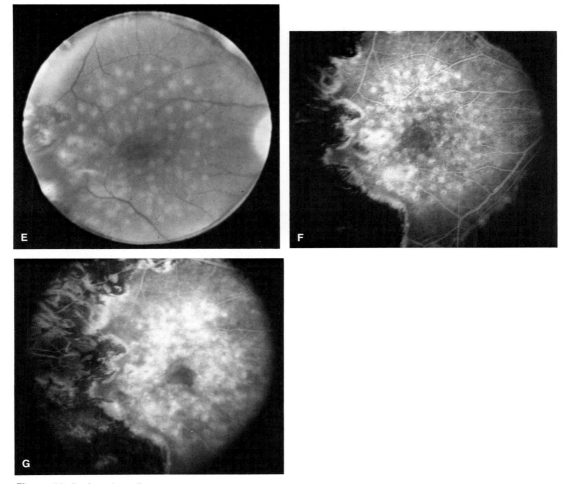

Figure 10–2 (continued)

COMBINED TREATMENT FOR MACULAR EDEMA AND PROLIFERATIVE RETINOPATHY

Peripheral panretinal photocoagulation for proliferative retinopathy has been associated with moderate visual loss after treatment, especially in eyes with preexisting macular edema.[19–26] This visual loss, although usually transient, has been partly attributed to exacerbation of the macular edema. It has been suggested that focal, or grid, treatment to diabetic macular edema may reduce this adverse macular effect of panretinal photocoagulation if initiated before peripheral panretinal photocoagulation, for instance, when proliferative retinopathy is less than high risk.[24–26]

The presence of both proliferative retinopathy and significant macular edema can be approached in any of several different ways. The macular edema can be treated first, if the proliferative retinopathy is not yet high risk, followed by panretinal photocoagulation when indicated. However, if the proliferative disease is either at or rapidly approaching the high-risk level, it must be treated expeditiously. The proliferative retinopathy may be treated first, followed by the treatment of macular edema; this may be accompanied by the known side effect

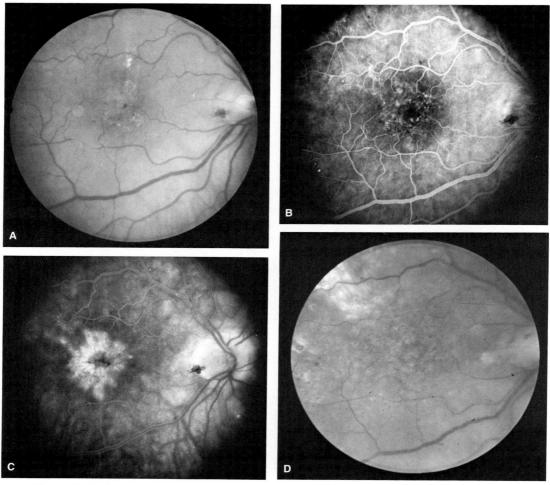

Figure 10–3 A 75-year-old white man, 2 months post-cataract–extraction with an IOL in his right eye, who has insulin-dependent diabetes of 12-years duration. Visual acuity was 20/200 on presentation. (**A**) He has nonproliferative diabetic retinopathy, macular thickening, and definite cysts seen on slit-lamp biomicroscopy. (**B**) On fluorescein angiography the irregular early capillary microaneurysmal changes were more consistent with diabetic maculopathy, and (**C**) a late frame of the angiogram shows leakage, confirming cystoid macular edema. Note that the hyperfluorescence seen around the optic disc is consistent with staining of the scleral crescent, but there is no leakage over the optic nerve itself and no postinflammatory hyperemia. The absence of leakage over the optic nerve, combined with the findings on the early frames of the angiogram, suggests that the macular edema in this patient is more likely diabetic in origin, rather than pseudophakic. He received modified grid treatment, after which visual acuity improved to 20/60 with (**D**) complete resolution of macular thickening and CME.

of panretinal photocoagulation—exacerbation of existing macular edema. Or, a combined treatment approach, as will be described in this section, can be used to treat both the proliferative disease and macular edema at the same time, without experiencing this side effect.[27]

Treatment Technique

After determining the presence of central macular edema and the presence of significant peripheral retinopathy during the clinical examination, a fluorescein angiogram is obtained to guide us in the pattern of macular treatment.

Either retrobulbar or peribulbar anesthesia of a 50:50 mixture of 0.75% bupivacaine and 2% lidocaine with hyaluronidase (Wydase) or topical anesthesia is used. Some patients, in our experience, tolerate the initial session better with the akinesia and anesthesia afforded by the injectable anesthetic. A recent fluorescein angiogram is projected during the macular treatment. In general, the same wavelength is used for both the macular and the peripheral treatments and at subsequent sessions. We generally prefer the argon green wavelength, although krypton red is useful in cases of media opacity, such as hemorrhage or dense cataract.

Patients receive the combined treatment in two sessions: in the first session, modified grid or focal treatment to the macula is combined with panretinal photocoagulation to the inferior half of the retina; this is followed 2 to 3 weeks later by completion of the panretinal photocoagulation to the superior half of the retina. In selected patients, the entire combined treatment is given in a single session; these circumstances include patients who have demonstrated prior noncompliance or have difficulty in returning for follow-up. The technique of modified grid[27–30] or focal treatment has previously been described (see Chapter 5). We first apply a posterior pole lens to the eye for the macular treatment. A panfunduscopic lens is then applied to perform the panretinal photocoagulation as described in Chapter 6. We set the laser delivery system at the 500-μm size for the panretinal photocoagulation, with the goal of 800 to 900 spots to the inferior half of the retina in the first session (Fig. 10-4). Two to three weeks later, an average of 900 spots is added in the second session to the superior one-half of the retina, completing the panretinal treatment (Figs. 10-5 through 10-7). Patients are asked to return in 6 to 8 weeks following completion of the combined treatment to assess their response to the panretinal photocoagulation. If there is no response or there is progression of the proliferative retinopathy, supplemental panretinal photocoagulation can be applied. Macular treatments are given supplementally at an interval of 3 to 4 months, and only if the central retina involving the foveal

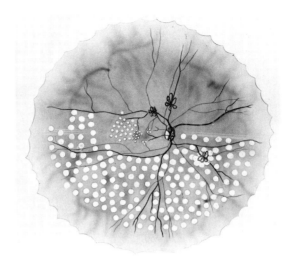

Figure 10–4 Artist's illustration. First session of combined treatment: macular treatment in modified grid or focal photocoagulation pattern is given first, followed by panretinal photocoagulation to the inferior one-half of the retina, with local treatment to the retina underlying flat surface NVE.

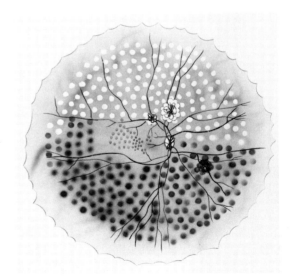

Figure 10–5 Artist's illustration. Second session of combined treatment: 2 to 3 weeks later, panretinal photocoagulation is completed by applying treatment to the superior one-half of the retina.

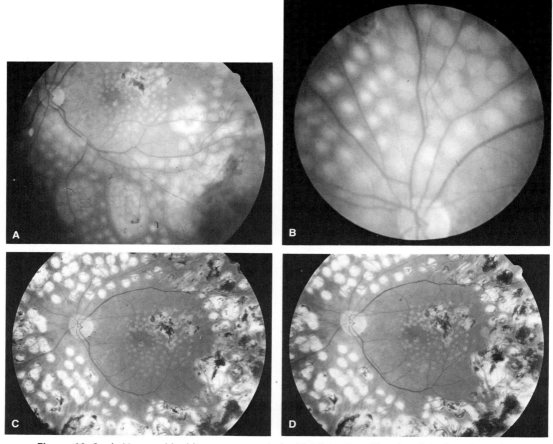

Figure 10–6   A 41-year-old white man presented with bilateral proliferative diabetic retinopathy, status post-focal treatment 5 years before presentation. (His left eye is presented here.) He was seen with proliferative diabetic retinopathy with high-risk retinopathy and preretinal hemorrhage, in addition to diffuse diabetic macular edema, particularly temporal to the fovea. (**A**) He received combined modified grid and panretinal photocoagulation to the inferior one-half retina, with confluent treatment applied to areas of NVE. (**B**) This was followed 2 weeks later by completion of panretinal photocoagulation to the superior one-half of the retina. (**C**) Two years and (**D**) 4 years posttreatment, there is complete regression of neovascularization and no evidence of recurrent macular edema.

avascular zone is still thickened on clinical biomicroscopic examination. We maintain the same parameters as used for supplemental macular or panretinal treatments (Fig. 10-8).

In our review of 52 eyes with both diffuse diabetic macular edema and proliferative retinopathy—both early and high risk—treated with combined macular modified grid and full peripheral panretinal photocoagulation either in one or two sessions, visual acuity was shown to improve in 4%, remain unchanged in 72%, and become worse in 24% of treated eyes

at 2 years. This is comparable with our results for eyes treated for diffuse diabetic macular edema alone.[28–30] We also noted that only 10% of eyes had lost three or more lines of vision compared with baseline at the 4- and 8-month follow-up visits after completion of combined treatment.[27] In the Diabetic Retinopathy Study (DRS), 26% of eyes with high-risk retinopathy and macular edema present at baseline demonstrated a visual loss of two or more lines at the 4-month follow-up when treated with pan-

(continued on page 168)

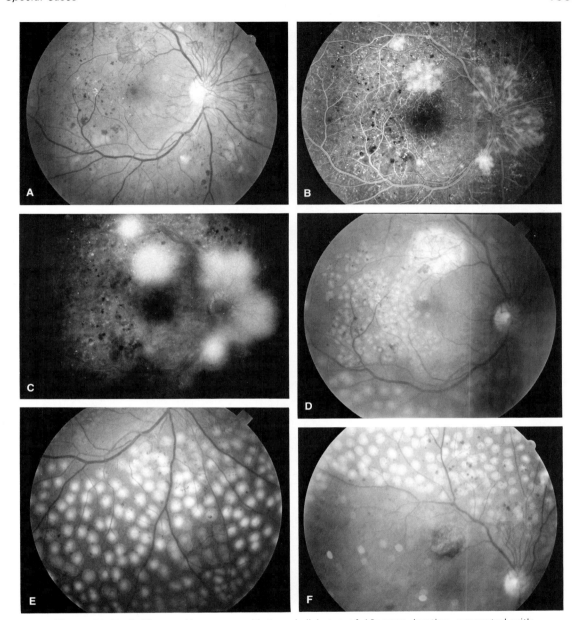

Figure 10–7 A 42-year-old woman, with type I diabetes of 10-years duration, presented with **(A–C)** high-risk retinopathy with extensive NVD, NVE, and diffuse diabetic macular edema. **(D,E)** Combined modified grid and panretinal photocoagulation treatment to the inferior one-half of the retina were performed, including confluent treatment to the retina underlying surface NVE located just inside the superotemporal arcade. This was followed 3 weeks later by **(F)** completion of the panretinal photocoagulation to the superior one-half retina. Visual acuity remained at 20/25 throughout follow-up.

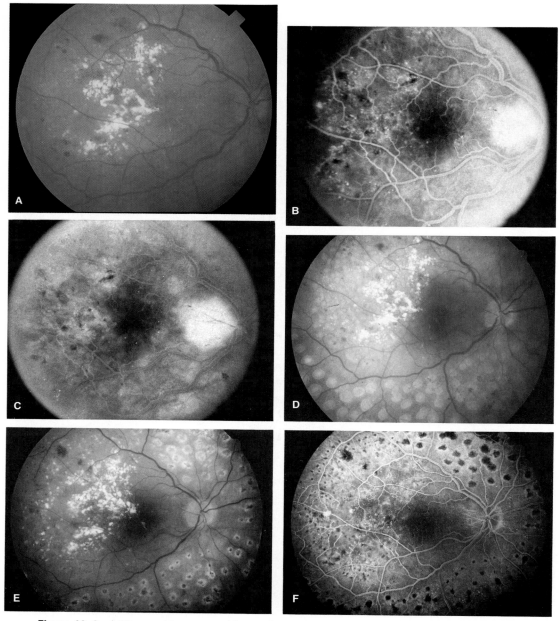

Figure 10–8   A 55-year-old woman, with type II diabetes of 15-years duration, presented with (**A**) diffuse exudative diabetic macular edema with high-risk retinopathy. (**B,C**) Fluorescein angiography revealed diffuse leakage in the perifoveal capillary network and leakage from the NVD. She underwent combined photocoagulation treatment with grid and panretinal photocoagulation in two sessions. (**D**) The first session is shown. (**E–G**) Her follow-up showed persistent diabetic macular edema, as well as persistent NVE with new preretinal hemorrhage inferiorly. (**H**) Supplemental modified grid and panretinal photocoagulation were given. Note that the new panretinal photocoagulation is placed in areas not previously treated. Six months after supplemental treatment, she had no evidence of proliferative disease, but (**I**) diabetic macular edema persisted, with new increased hard exudate centrally, and (**J,K**) diffuse leakage with cystic changes, as shown in the late frames of the fluorescein angiogram. (**L**) She received a second supplemental modified grid treatment. Six months later, residual islands of edema were present temporal to the macula. (**M**) Temporal islands of macular edema remained but the central macular edema involving the foveal avascular zone had resolved. Therefore, no additional modified grid treatment was recommended and (**N**) 1 year later the central macula remained flat. Visual acuity remained stable at 20/80.

(continued)

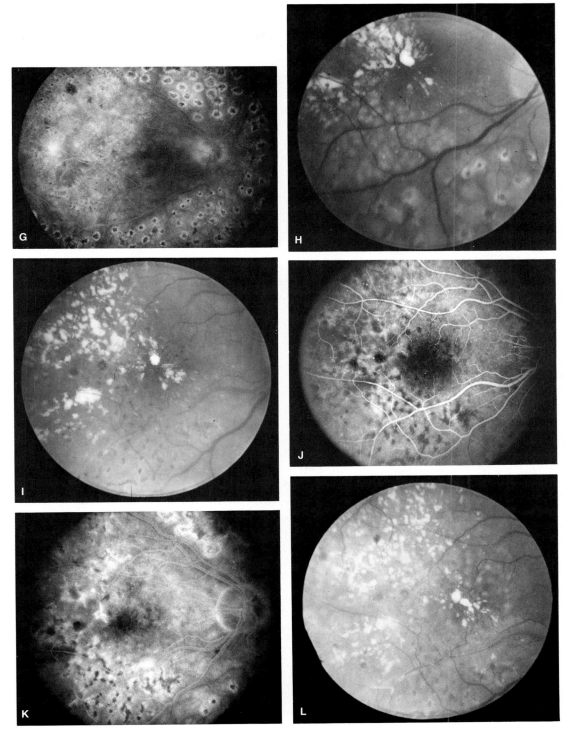

Figure 10–8 (continued)

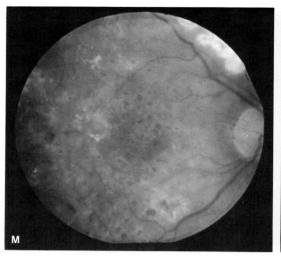 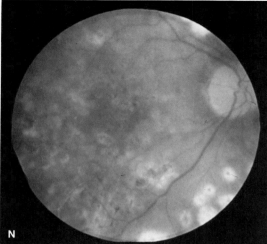

Figure 10–8   (continued)

retinal photocoagulation alone.[31] Twenty-eight percent of eyes in another study, followed for less than 1 year after panretinal photocoagulation, experienced a loss of two or more lines of vision.[22] Although our study was not directly comparable with the DRS or other previous reports, we believe that the reduction in visual loss—especially in the early follow-up visits—reflects a beneficial effect of the concurrent macular treatment and allows more eyes to retain their initial visual acuity (Fig. 10-9).

In one strategy of the Early Treatment Diabetic Retinopathy Study (ETDRS), eyes with severe nonproliferative or early proliferative diabetic retinopathy and macular edema were randomized to one of four protocols in the early-treatment group, including immediate full-scatter and focal treatment.[26] It is not explicitly stated whether focal and scatter treatments were performed at the same session or within a short interval of time. This strategy was shown to be efficacious in reducing the rate of severe visual loss, but, as we have previously discussed, all rates of severe visual loss in this study were low. Overall, early photocoagulation had a beneficial effect in reducing moderate visual loss in the long term. Although full scatter, despite macular treatment, appeared to be associated with some degree of early moderate visual loss compared with deferral, the relatively reduced rates of moderate

visual loss overall in eyes with macular edema were attributed to the beneficial effects of macular treatment.

In eyes with severe nonproliferative or early proliferative retinopathy and coexistent significant macular edema, one may choose to treat the peripheral disease either at the same time or before or even following the treatment of the macula.[26] However, as the risk of progression to high-risk retinopathy is substantial for certain subsets of severe nonproliferative (for instance, when an eye has two of the three characteristics in the 4-2-1 rule) or early proliferative disease,[32] careful and meticulous follow-up of the proliferative disease must be maintained to assure appropriate and timely intervention if it is chosen to follow the peripheral disease. If, based on clinical judgment, it is decided that early panretinal photocoagulation will be initiated, we recommend treating both the macular edema and the proliferative disease in our combined treatment approach.

DIABETIC RETINOPATHY IN PREGNANCY

All diabetic patients who become pregnant should have a baseline dilated fundus examination in their first trimester, since it is agreed

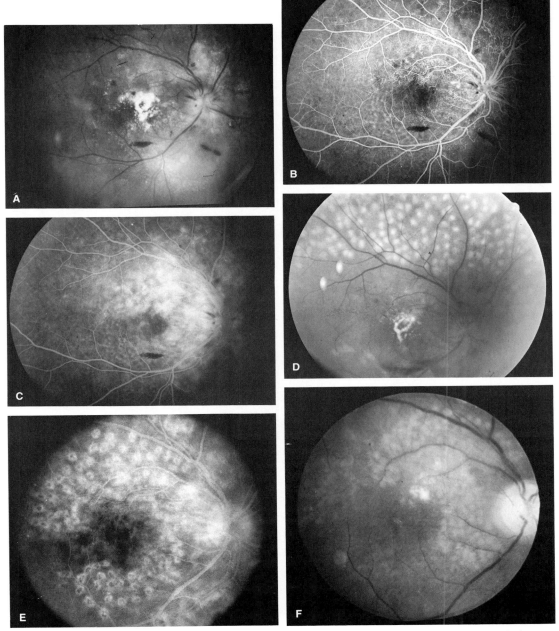

Figure 10–9 A 25-year-old white woman presented 6 months postpartum with (**A–C**) preretinal hemorrhage and NVD, with massive exudative maculopathy and diffuse diabetic macular edema. Visual acuity was 20/200. The patient underwent combined panretinal photocoagulation and modified grid treatment for macular edema in two sessions. Three months later the neovascularization on the disc showed no regression and new preretinal hemorrhage was present inferiorly. (**D**) Supplemental panretinal photocoagulation was given at that time. Visual acuity was 20/70. Six months later new diffuse diabetic macular edema was noted and (**E**) the late-frame fluorescein angiogram showed diffuse leakage. (**F**) Supplemental modified grid treatment was performed. (**G**) Four months later, she had persistent diffuse diabetic macular edema and (**H**) received another supplemental modified grid treatment. Visual acuity was 20/40. Nine months later, (**I**) there was resolution of the central macular edema with complete resorption of her macular exudate and (**J**) complete resolution of her proliferative disease. Visual acuity was 20/40.

(continued)

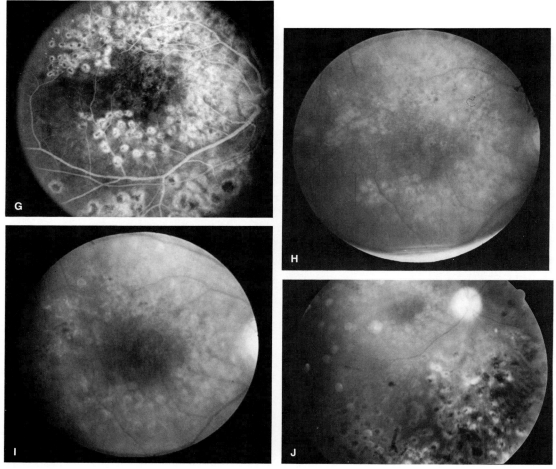

Figure 10–9 (continued)

that pregnancy can accelerate diabetic retinopathy.[33–37] This may be simply a reflection of the relative duration of diabetes present in pregnant diabetic women, since most of these patients of childbearing age will have had insulin-dependent diabetes for at least 5 years or more.[33,34] Or there may be factors, both metabolic and hormonal, that contribute to the overall deterioration of retinopathy in the pregnant patient (Fig. 10-10).

Patients with either no or minimal retinopathy before pregnancy will generally carry out their gestational period with only minimal new changes in their retinopathy and only rarely will have visually significant changes. Of patients with mild nonproliferative retinopathy at the beginning of pregnancy, up to 47% have

been shown to develop progressive amounts of changes up through what would now be considered moderate-to-severe nonproliferative retinopathy.[33,34,36,37] Only 5% of these patients progress to proliferative retinopathy.[37] However, 46% of patients who start pregnancy with any proliferative retinopathy will progressively develop worse retinopathy if left untreated.[37]

Patients with changes consistent with mild nonproliferative retinopathy have been shown to have acceleration of their retinopathy in the second trimester and may show spontaneous improvement by term and postpartum.[33,34] Although such reversible changes have been reported[33,34,38] whereby diabetic retinopathy has been demonstrated to even regress spontaneously postpartum, we recommend that

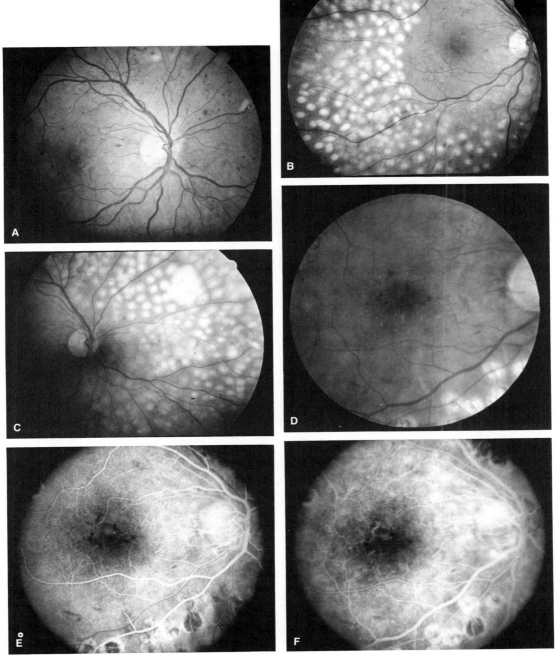

Figure 10–10 A 20-year-old juvenile-onset insulin-dependent diabetic presented with (**A**) high-risk proliferative diabetic retinopathy in her right eye. (**B,C**) She underwent two sessions of panretinal photocoagulation in the next month, and required two additional sessions of panretinal photocoagulation to stabilize her proliferative disease. However, (**D**) she developed diffuse diabetic macular edema 18 months after her initial presentation, (**E,F**) confirmed on fluorescein angiography. (**G**) Modified grid photocoagulation was performed. (**H,I**) Four months later she had no residual macular edema, and (**J**) there was no residual proliferative disease. Note the appearance of the optic disc and regression of NVD. One year later, when she was 3 months pregnant, she presented (**K**) with new NVD along the inferior margin of the disc with preretinal hemorrhage. She was treated with supplemental panretinal photocoagulation. No recurrence of the hemorrhage was noted and she delivered a healthy baby by cesarean section. (**L,M**) Six months after delivery, her retinopathy was stable with no evidence of recurrence of either her proliferative or macular disease.

(continued)

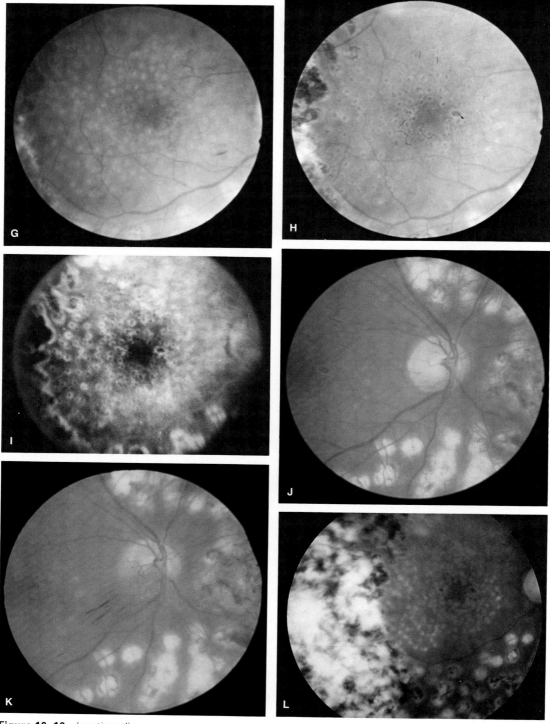

Figure 10–10 (continued)

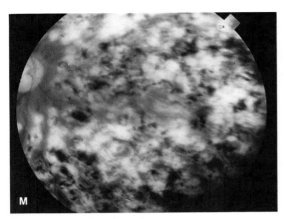

Figure 10–10   (continued)

pregnant patients who are seen with retinopathy of the very severe nonproliferative grade or worse be considered for early photocoagulation treatment before development of high-risk characteristics. The response to panretinal photocoagulation appears to be similar to that of nonpregnant patients[39,40] (Fig. 10-11).

We recommend that all pregnant diabetic patients be checked at the beginning of their pregnancy and during each trimester; the frequency of follow-up is determined by the initial findings on the baseline examination.[41] Patients seen with mild nonproliferative changes should be followed at least once each trimester, and patients with more severe retinopathy more frequently, with the goal of early intervention.

Macular edema has also been noted to worsen during pregnancy.[35] Macular edema left untreated has been shown to either regress spontaneously postpartum or to worsen, causing substantial visual loss. It is often noted with a concurrent increase in peripheral retinopathy.[35] Although clinical evidence is sufficient to determine both the presence of macular edema and proliferative retinopathy, we generally require fluorescein angiography in the nonpregnant diabetic patient to guide us in the pattern of macular photocoagulation. However, the use of fluorescein angiography during pregnancy is generally avoided, except for potential sight-threatening conditions, such as choroidal neovascular membranes.

There have been no teratogenic or embryocidal effects in animal studies to our knowledge,[37,42–44] and a recent review by Halperin and coauthors[45] found no higher rate of birth anomalies or complications when fluorescein angiography was used during pregnancy. However, we do not perform fluorescein angiography for the purpose of treating diabetic macular edema during pregnancy, as the safety of fluorescein angiography has yet to be demonstrated conclusively.[45–47] If macular edema is noted on slit-lamp biomicroscopic examination, we follow the patient clinically until term. Approximately 3 to 4 months after delivery, fluorescein angiography can be obtained safely, and appropriate treatment can be given with laser photocoagulation (as described in Chapter 5). The peripheral retinopathy is treated, as is customary, with panretinal photocoagulation, based strictly on our clinical findings.

Our recommendations for follow-up are concerned with pregnant patients with a known history of diabetes. Patients with gestational diabetes do not appear to be at risk for the exacerbation of retinopathy.[33,37]

Lastly, earlier reports associating an unacceptably high rate of fetal death and congenital abnormalities with severity of retinopathy[48,49] are no longer applicable. The advances made in the prenatal care of a pregnant diabetic patient, both in her metabolic and ophthalmologic care, have improved the outcomes of both the mother and the fetus during pregnancy.[37,50] Although it has been suggested that strict metabolic control initiated during pregnancy may, in and of itself, be associated with at least a temporary worsening of retinopathy,[36] this practice has contributed to the overall well being of both the mother and fetus,[37,50] and is currently recommended.

THE ADVANCED CASES

We refer to eyes with diabetic macular edema, macular ischemia as seen on the fluorescein angiogram, and visual acuity of less than 20/80

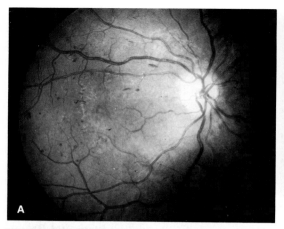

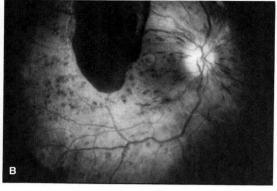

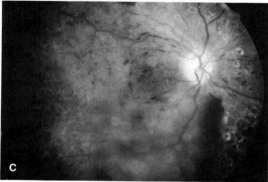

Figure 10–11 A 28-year-old white woman, with a 21-year history of insulin-dependent diabetes, presented with (**A**) nonproliferative diabetic retinopathy in her right eye. Six months later she returned in her first trimester of pregnancy with (**B**) proliferative diabetic retinopathy and preretinal and subhyaloid hemorrhage. She received panretinal photocoagulation immediately, with gradual resorption of blood and involution of her proliferative diabetic retinopathy during her pregnancy. (**C**) Fundus photographs 1 month post-panretinal photocoagulation showed some resorption of hemorrhage. Five years after initial treatment, she has minimal fibrotic changes along the inferotemporal arcade, without evidence of proliferative diabetic retinopathy. She was followed closely, but no additional treatment was required during the course of her pregnancy.

as the advanced cases. We are unaware of any specific report studying the efficacy of treatment on this subset of patients. When we review the fluorescein angiogram before treatment for macular edema, we examine the state of the perifoveal capillary bed, looking specifically in part for the amount of capillary dropout or remodeling of the capillary bed.[51,52] In addition, we attempt to quantify the size of the foveal avascular zone. Since we feel that the amount of ischemia is not necessarily predictive of the ultimate visual outcome, we have looked at 80 consecutive cases of diffuse diabetic macular edema with moderate capillary nonperfusion, quantifying the amount of ischemia by clock hours of dropout (unpublished data). From our preliminary results we have found that unless severe capillary nonperfusion exists, with "wipeout" of the perifoveal capillary bed, the visual results of these advanced eyes treated with modified grid photocoagulation are comparable with the results

of eyes treated for diffuse diabetic macular edema alone (Fig. 10-12).

Currently, unless an eye has capillary wipeout, or if we feel that photocoagulation treatment will eliminate the last few vessels of capillary perfusion to the macula, we recommend that all eyes with clinical evidence of central retinal thickening be considered for photocoagulation treatment, the pattern of treatment being dependent on the type of leakage seen on the angiogram (Fig. 10-13). However, since most eyes in this particular series had a preoperative visual acuity of 20/80 or worse and that over 70% of eyes retained their preoperative vision without change, this level of vision may also represent the natural course of an eye with macular ischemia. In other words, had these eyes not been treated, they might not have lost any further vision, but rather, remained at that same relatively poor level.[53] We also do not exclude patients with eyes that have substantial exudate, as we have clinically

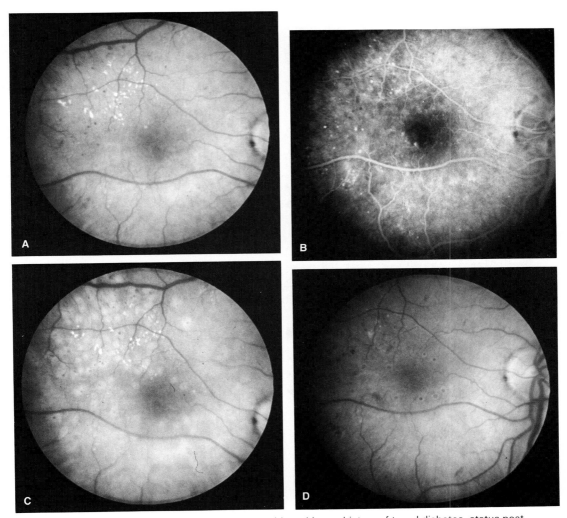

Figure 10–12 A 66-year-old white woman, with an 11-year history of type I diabetes, status post-extracapsular cataract extraction 7 years earlier, presented with visual acuity of 20/40 and (**A**) diffuse diabetic macular edema. (**B**) On fluorescein angiography, she had an irregular and enlarged parafoveal capillary network and diffuse leakage, primarily temporal and superotemporal to the FAZ. (**C**) Modified grid laser photocoagulation was applied to areas of retinal thickening superotemporally as well as to individual leaking microaneurysms around and temporal to the FAZ. (**D,E**) Four months later, she had residual thickening and (**F**) supplemental modified grid laser was applied temporal to the FAZ (**G**). Eighteen months after initial treatment, she had no residual retinal thickening and her visual acuity was 20/16. (**H**) Four years later her visual acuity was stable at 20/25.

(continued)

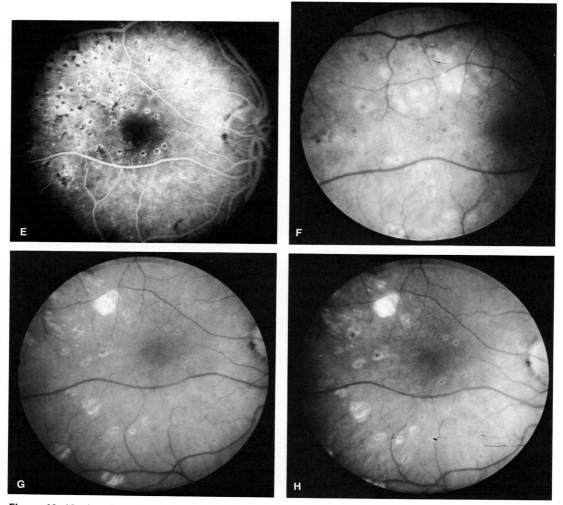

Figure 10–12   (continued)

seen many cases that have presented with thick exudative maculopathy and have shown a favorable response to macular treatment (Fig. 10-14).

DIABETIC OR HYPERTENSIVE RETINOPATHY

Hypertensive retinal changes are commonly seen in the older nondiabetic and diabetic population. These include arteriolar narrowing, retinal microaneurysms, cotton-wool spots, arteriolosclerotic changes of the vessel walls,

and arteriolovenous "nicking."[54,55] The overlapping findings with diabetic retinopathy can be somewhat confusing, especially in a state of accelerated hypertension. Patients will generally complain of rapid visual loss. Numerous retinal hemorrhages, especially flame-shaped hemorrhages of the nerve fiber layer, and cotton-wool spots are seen within the posterior pole and appear to emanate from the optic nerve head. Large amounts of exudate can be seen and will look like a star if located in the macula.

Ischemic changes to the vessel walls will cause leakage of fluorescein or staining of the vessel walls. Numerous patches of nonperfu-

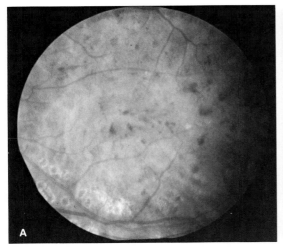

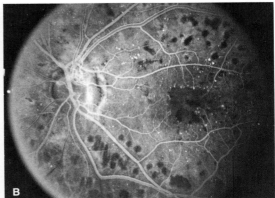

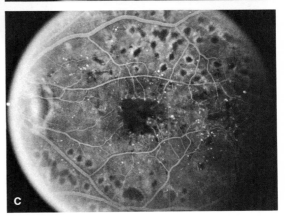

Figure 10–13 A 55-year-old man, status post-panretinal photocoagulation for proliferative retinopathy, with a history of recent visual loss decrease to 20/200, presented with (**A**) mild retinal thickening primarily temporal to the FAZ, and (**B,C**) fluorescein angiography showed marked enlargement of the FAZ with macular ischemia. Because of this and because no central thickening was present, macular photocoagulation was not recommended for this patient.

sion can be seen angiographically owing to fibrinoid necrosis of the choriocapillaris and large choroidal vessels.[55] Localized neurosensory detachments may be noted, caused by damage to the normal retinal pigment epithelial cell function, secondary to the necrosis of the choriocapillaris.[55] Accelerated hypertension can cause optic nerve head swelling, with dilation of the capillaries supplying the disc; with fluorescein angiography, the optic nerve head will appear hyperfluorescent, with leakage from the dilated capillaries.

All of these changes distinguish hypertensive retinopathy from that which is primarily diabetic; we look at the configuration of the vessels and the location and amount of intraretinal hemorrhages, cotton-wool spots, and exudate. Most importantly, we check for a history of hypertension and measure the actual blood pressure at the time of examination (Fig. 10-15).

MONOCULAR PATIENT OR POOR FELLOW EYE

If a patient is either anatomically or functionally monocular, it is incumbent upon the treating ophthalmologist to provide as efficacious and timely treatment as possible to the remaining eye. Early panretinal photocoagulation should be considered for severe or very severe nonproliferative or early proliferative disease in the monocular patient to try to prevent the sequelae of proliferative disease and the higher risk of severe visual loss when treated after reaching three retinopathy risk factors or high-risk retinopathy. The patient should be advised of the potential loss of peripheral visual field and other psychophysical parameters. In an only eye with early significant macular edema with excellent vision, we tend to be more conservative. We will elect to follow the patient until the time when the edema either worsens

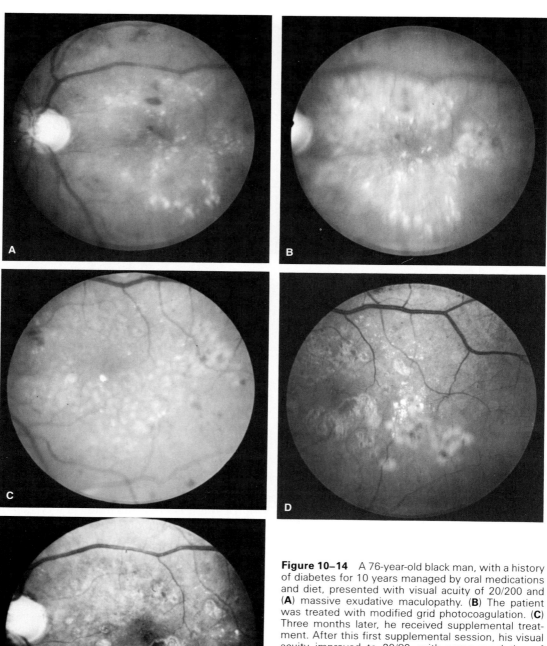

Figure 10–14 A 76-year-old black man, with a history of diabetes for 10 years managed by oral medications and diet, presented with visual acuity of 20/200 and (**A**) massive exudative maculopathy. (**B**) The patient was treated with modified grid photocoagulation. (**C**) Three months later, he received supplemental treatment. After this first supplemental session, his visual acuity improved to 20/80, with some resolution of macular edema, but (**D**) required a second supplemental laser treatment for residual central thickening. Three years after presentation, having had three modified grid treatments, the patient had complete resolution of his exudative maculopathy. (**E**) The central macula is flat, and visual acuity is 20/30.

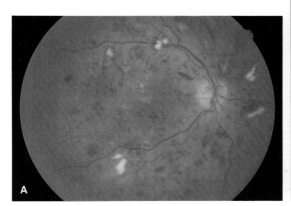
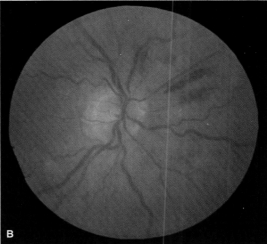

Figure 10–15   A 65-year-old man came to the emergency room complaining of sudden visual loss during the preceding 24 hours. He had a history of non–insulin-dependent diabetes of 5 years duration. (**A**) Examination revealed numerous nerve fiber layer hemorrhages and intraretinal hemorrhages, with cotton-wool spots scattered throughout the posterior pole and all four quadrants. (**B**) There was no evidence of proliferative disease. His blood pressure was 280/180 and his fundus findings suggested primarily hypertensive retinopathy.

or the vision begins to drop slightly, to avoid the potential paracentral scotomas that can accompany macular photocoagulation treatment. If the central macula is thickened clinically and the fluorescein angiogram reveals an acceptable amount of perfusion, we will advocate macular photocoagulation. In the patient with only one functional eye, reliable and frequent follow-up with early intervention is the mainstay of preventing visual loss resulting from the complications of diabetic retinopathy.

References

1. National Society to Prevent Blindness, Operational Research Department. Vision problems in the US: a statistical analysis. New York: National Society to Prevent Blindness, 1980:1–46.
2. Javitt JC, Aiello LP, Bassi LJ, et al. Detecting and treating retinopathy in patients with type I diabetes mellitus. Ophthalmology 1991; 98:1565–1574.
3. Klein R, Klein BEK, Moss SE, Davis MD, DeMets DL. The Wisconsin Epidemiologic Study of Diabetic Retinopathy. II. Prevalence and risk of diabetic retinopathy when age at diagnosis is less than 30 years. Arch Ophthalmol 1984; 102:520–526.
4. Klein R, Klein BEK, Moss SE, Davis MD, DeMets DL. The Wisconsin Epidemiologic Study of Diabetic Retinopathy. III. Prevalence and risk of diabetic retinopathy when age at diagnosis is 30 or more years. Arch Ophthalmol 1984; 102:527–532.
5. Klein R, Klein BEK, Moss SE, Davis MD, DeMets DL. The Wisconsin Epidemiologic Study of Diabetic Retinopathy. IX. Four-year incidence and progression of diabetic retinopathy when age at diagnosis is less than 30 years. Arch Ophthalmol 1989; 107:237–243.
6. Klein R, Klein BEK, Moss SE, Davis MD, DeMets DL. The Wisconsin Epidemiologic Study of Diabetic Retinopathy. X. Four-year incidence and progression of diabetic retinopathy when age at diagnosis is 30 years or more. Arch Ophthalmol 1989; 107:244–249.
7. Klein, R. The epidemiology of diabetic retinopathy: findings from the Wisconsin Epidemiologic Study of Diabetic Retinopathy. Int Ophthalmol Clin 1987; 27:230–238.
8. Klein R, Klein BEK, Moss SE, Davis MD, DeMets DL. The Wisconsin Epidemiologic Study of Diabetic Retinopathy. IV. Diabetic macular edema. Ophthalmology 1984; 91:1464–1474.
9. Klein R, Klein BEK, Moss SE, Davis MD, DeMets DL. The Wisconsin Epidemiologic Study of Diabetic Retinopathy. XI. The incidence of macular edema. Ophthalmology 1989; 96:1501–1510.
10. Gass JDM. Retinal capillary disease. In: Stereoscopic atlas of macular diseases. St. Louis: CV Mosby Co; 1987:368–373.
11. Aiello LM, Wand M, Liang G. Neovascular glaucoma and vitreous hemorrhage following cataract surgery in patients with diabetes mellitus. Am Acad Ophthalmol 1984; 90:814–820.
12. Poliner LS, Christianson DJ, Escoffery RF, Kolker AE,

Gordon ME. Neovascular glaucoma after intracapsular and extracapsular cataract extraction in diabetic patients. Am J Ophthalmol 1985; 100:637–643.

13. Rice TA, Michels RG. Long term anatomic and functional results of vitrectomy for diabetic retinopathy. Am J Ophthalmol 1980; 90:297–303.

14. Blankenship GW. The lens influence on diabetic vitrectomy results. Arch Ophthalmol 1980; 98:2196–2198.

15. Rice TA, Michels RG, Maguire MG, Rice EF. The effect of lensectomy on the incidence of iris neovascularization and neovascular glaucoma after vitrectomy for diabetic retinopathy. Am J Ophthalmol 1983; 95:1–11.

16. Blankenship GW, Flynn HW, Kokame GT. Posterior chamber intraocular lens insertion during pars plana lensectomy and vitrectomy for complications of proliferative diabetic retinopathy. Am J Ophthalmol 1989; 108:1–5.

17. Gass JDM, Norton EWD. Cystoid macular edema and papilledema following cataract extraction: a fluorescein funduscopic and angiographic study. Arch Ophthalmol 1966; 76:646–661.

18. Stark WJ Jr, Maumenee AE, Fagadau W, et al. Cystoid macular edema in pseudophakia. Surv Ophthalmol 1984; 28:442–451.

19. Diabetic Retinopathy Study Research Group. Photocoagulation treatment of proliferative diabetic retinopathy: the second report of diabetic retinopathy/vitrectomy study findings. Am J Ophthalmol 1978; 85:82–106.

20. Meyers SM. Macular edema after scatter laser photocoagulation for proliferative diabetic retinopathy. Am J Ophthalmol 1980; 90:210–216.

21. McDonald HR, Schatz H. Macular edema following panretinal photocoagulation. Retina 1985; 5:5–10.

22. McDonald HR, Schatz H. Visual loss following panretinal photocoagulation for proliferative diabetic retinopathy. Ophthalmology 1985; 92:388–393.

23. Blankenship GW. A clinical comparison of central and peripheral argon laser panretinal photocoagulation for proliferative diabetic retinopathy. Ophthalmology 1988; 95:170–177.

24. Ferris FL, Podgor MJ, Davis MD, The Diabetic Retinopathy Study Research Group. Report no 12. Macular edema in diabetic retinopathy study patients. Ophthalmology 1987; 94:754–760.

25. Kleiner RC, Elman MJ, Murphy RP, Ferris FL III. Transient severe visual loss after panretinal photocoagulation. Am J Ophthalmol 1988; 106:298–306.

26. Early Treatment Diabetic Retinopathy Study Research Group. Report no 9. Early photocoagulation for diabetic retinopathy. Ophthalmology 1991; 98:766–785.

27. Lee CM, Olk RJ. Combined modified grid and panretinal photocoagulation for diffuse diabetic macular edema and proliferative retinopathy. Presented at the 1991 meeting of the Am Acad of Ophthalmol (submitted for publication).

28. Olk RJ. Modified grid argon (blue-green) laser photocoagulation for diffuse macular edema. Ophthalmology 1986; 93:938–950.

29. Olk RJ. Argon green (514 nm) versus krypton red (647 nm) modified grid laser photocoagulation for diffuse diabetic macular edema. Ophthalmology 1990; 97:1101–1113.

30. Lee CM, Olk RJ. Modified grid laser photocoagulation for diffuse diabetic macular edema: long-term visual results. Ophthalmology 1991; 98:1594–1602.

31. Diabetic Retinopathy Study Research Group. Report no 14. Indication for photocoagulation treatment of diabetic retinopathy. Int Ophthalmol Clin 1987; 27:239–252.

32. Early Treatment Diabetic Retinopathy Study Research Group. Report no 12. Fundus photographic risk factors for progression of diabetic retinopathy. Ophthalmology 1991; 98:823–833.

33. Horvat M, Maclean H, Goldberg L, Crock GW. Diabetic retinopathy in pregnancy: a 12-year prospective survey. Br J Ophthalmol 1980; 64:398–403.

34. Moloney JB, Drury MI. The effect of pregnancy on the natural course of diabetic retinopathy. Am J Ophthalmol 1982; 93:745–756.

35. Sinclair SH, Nesler C, Foxman B, Nichols CW, Gabbe S. Macular edema and pregnancy in insulin-dependent diabetes. Am J Ophthalmol 1984; 97:154–167.

36. Phelps RL, Sakor P, Metzger BE, Jampol L, Freinkel N. Changes in diabetic retinopathy during pregnancy. Arch Ophthalmol 1986; 104:1806–1810.

37. Sunness JS. The pregnant woman's eye. Surv Ophthalmol 1988; 32:219–238.

38. Ohrt V. The influence of pregnancy on diabetic retinopathy with special regard to the reversible changes shown in 100 pregnancies. Acta Ophthalmol 1984; 62:603–616.

39. Johnston GP. Pregnancy and diabetic retinopathy. Am J Ophthalmol 1980; 90: 519–524.

40. Hercules BL, Wozencroft M, Gayed II, Jeacock J. Peripheral retinal ablation in the treatment of proliferative diabetic retinopathy during pregnancy. Br J Ophthalmol 1980; 64:87–93.

41. American Academy of Ophthalmology. Preferred practice pattern. Diabetic retinopathy. San Francisco: American Academy of Ophthalmology; 1989.

42. Shirai S, Majima A. Effects of fluorescein-sodium injected to mother mice on the embryo. Folia Ophthalmol Jpn 1975; 26:132–137.

43. McEnery JK, Wong WP, Peyman GA. Evaluation of the teratogenicity of fluorescein sodium. Am J Ophthalmol 1977; 84:847–850.

44. Salem H, Loux JJ, Smith S, et al. Evaluation of the toxicologic and teratogenic potentials of sodium fluorescein in the rat. Toxicology 1979; 12:143–150.

45. Halperin LS, Olk RJ, Soubrane G, et al. Safety of fluorescein angiography during pregnancy. Am J Ophthalmol 1990; 109:563–566.

46. Greenberg F, Lewis RA. Safety of fluorescein angiog-

raphy during pregnancy [Letter]: Halperin LS, Olk RJ, Soubrane G, et al. Reply. Am J Ophthalmol 1990; 110:323–325.

47. Yannuzzi LA, Roher KT, Tindel LJ, et al. Fluorescein angiography complication survey. Ophthalmology 1986; 93:611.

48. Beethan WP. Diabetic retinopathy in pregnancy. Trans Am Ophthalmol Soc 1950; 48:205–219.

49. White P. Pregnancy and diabetes, medical aspects. Med Clin North Am 1965; 49:1015–1024.

50. Frienkel N, Dooley SL, Metzger BE. Care of the pregnant woman with insulin-dependent diabetes. N Engl J Med 1985; 313:96–101.

51. Bresnick GH, Engerman R, Davis MD, et al. Patterns of ischemia in diabetic retinopathy. Trans Am Acad Ophthalmol Otolaryngol 1976; 81:694.

52. Bresnick GH, Condit R, Syrjala S, Palta M, Groo A, Korth K. Abnormalities of the foveal avascular zone in diabetic retinopathy. Arch Ophthalmol 1984; 102:1286–1293.

53. Ticho U, Patz A. The role of capillary perfusion in the management of diabetic macular edema. Am J Ophthalmol 1973; 76:880–886.

54. Ashton N. The eye in malignant hypertension. Trans Am Acad Ophthalmol Otolaryngol 1972; 76:17–40.

55. Tso MOM, Jampol LM. Pathophysiology of hypertensive retinopathy. Ophthalmologica 1982; 89:1132.

INDEX

Page numbers followed by *f* indicate illustrations; *t* following a page number indicates tabular material.

ISBN 0-397-51167-1